Suddenly Skinny Day by Day

A Weight Loss Memoir

Freya Taylor

Copyright © 2010-2012 Freya Taylor

All rights reserved.

ISBN: 1470113341
ISBN-13: 978-1470113346

CONTENTS

	Introduction	i
1	April	1
2	May	7
3	June	23
4	July	37
5	August	55
6	September	59
7	October	67
8	November	73
9	December	77
10	January	89
11	Transition	101

INTRODUCTION

I lost 100 pounds and 18 inches off my waist, in 9 months and 25 days. It was quite the roller-coaster adventure, as you can imagine. I wrote a book about surviving dramatic weight loss and all the radical life-changes it brings: *Suddenly Skinny*. This companion volume contains my journal entries from the first year of my journey. It details the daily ups and downs of remaining on plan – "OP." It contains my insights about weight loss, addiction to food, and managing my psyche.

I hope it can help you know you're not alone. Or at the very least, to know that you're not as crazy as I am.

1 APRIL

April 23: Waiting to start

My first food shipment arrives on Wednesday, or maybe Thursday. UPS always seems to show up at our offices at 8pm even though I put the business name on my shipments, so I may have to wait until Thursday to start.

I'm having dim sum with a big group next Saturday, I have family drama going on, and my law school exams start in 12 days. And yet, I will be starting this frickin' diet the moment the box shows up in my world. I am so over being fat! I don't care if it's convenient, or if I'm going to be spaced out and hungry during study days, or any of it. I just want to start clearing this off me.

I have been taking full advantage of my last few days of freedom. I want to be sure I have no regrets once I'm trying to make paste taste good for 6 months or so. I'll probably gain a couple more pounds by Wednesday, but, well, sometimes the little kid inside just needs a last can of Pringles for the road.

I picked Medifast [a meal replacement diet plan] because I work full time and do law school at night. I've had great success with South Beach before, but dear God I don't have time to be cooking that much fresh food right now. I can manage to cook once a week most weeks, and if food won't last until the next week it's takeout for me. So Medifast combines the upside of quick results with the absolutely required ease and portability.

I'm obsessively checking the tracking info and reading stuff on the Medifast site. I'm ready. Pass me the onion rings.

April 24: really focusing on noticing where I'm starting from

Day –4 or –5, depending on when my first box arrives.

Last night I was feeling anxious and stressed, and when I decided to go make some chili dip to eat with Tostitos, I felt the most lovely wave of relief. Just goodness. I don't usually let myself really notice the feelings that go with emotional eating, but I'm working on taking a fearless moral inventory of my fatness and the reasons for it. Eating the chili felt even better than deciding to eat it, and the overall sense of "it's all okay" persisted for quite a while, with my full belly.

I made a list of all the unpleasant things I experience with being so big, and I have it posted next to my list of goals and motivations. I want to capture all in one place the reasons why I want to do this. I'll start feeling better after a while, and begin thinking I can justify cheating, and I want to have a Very Clear snapshot of just what I'm leaving behind and why.

I feel like I've been struggling to hold up a huge weight for so long. I mean, literally I have been, as I'm carrying 100 pounds more than my frame is built to carry. But I always feel like I should make myself do things, go out, be social, get something accomplished, eat better, exercise, blah blah blah. I have such a long list of ways in which I tell myself I fail. I'm just tired all the time, and I don't feel festive or social or fun, I really don't.

Right now I'm letting it all go for a last few days. I'm not going and doing the social things I could be doing this weekend. My body doesn't want to, I don't feel like it, and I'm not going to force myself. I'm eating things that are not good for me, and just noticing how I feel when I do. I feel so good! I'm going to have to learn how to create that feeling in other ways, without food, and it's going to take a while. I'm trying to bookmark, notice, notice, bring into awareness, bring into consciousness, notice...

And relax. A few days of a fairly willpower-free zone. Then lots of it all at once.

Preparing, too. I inventoried my stores of Omega 3s and acidophilous. Have both. Bought Pam and Butter Buds and some

seasoned salts—I'm a little freaked out by the thought of powdered eggs but I shall do my best to get through it.
The overeater's relief. Sweet peace of a full belly. I'm going to miss that, a lot, and it's going to be damn hard to retrain those places. I am very glad I've decided it's time to do it, though.

April 25: Fearless and Searching Moral Inventory

Of where I'm starting from... I made a list. A long list. Of all the things I experience as unpleasant about being this fat. It includes the usual assortment of joint and back pain, displeasure with being unable to wear my closet-full of cute high heels, frustration with not enjoying dancing any more, etc. But I just want to share that the single-most horrifying thing about my body, today, is that I have a fat pad in the hollow of my throat. This is not a place on the human body that should collect a noticeable little bubble of fat.
Just not.

April 27: photos added!

I took "before" pics last night. Of course, they're "right now" pics at the moment. I feel a couple things about them—gently horrified at my complete lack of a waist and overall blocky rotund shape, and at the same time—excited to have these really awesome zomg fat before pics.
It's going to be so cool when I can start putting "afters" next to them.

April 28: UPS BRING ME MY BOX!!!!!!!!!!!!!!!!!!!!

I'm so eager to start I can't stand it! The box is "out for delivery" which could mean anytime, or even tomorrow, if they come after our offices close.
UPS, I'm begging you, don't make me go get real food for lunch. Let me eat a mint chocolate bar or oatmeal or chicken noodle soup, puhleeeze! [The Medifast food plan includes a lot of packets of diet versions of soups, oatmeal, pudding, shakes, etc.]

This fatty mcfatty is SO ready to start seeing the scale change (in the downward direction, of course!) On the upside, the last few days of "if I want it I can have it so I will be able to remember some final indulgences" has not resulted in any gain. Naughty foods, but not in such great quantity as to bump me up.

UPS!!!!!!!!!!!!!!!!!!!!!!!!!!!!!!!!

April 28: Panic sets in

My box arrived. Wow, are those some light, tiny, adorable, dollhouse-sized portions in those baggies. I must have gotten the child-sized box by mistake, right? For three-year-olds?

I should call them right away to see if I can get a replacement shipment. "Hello, Medifast? There's some mistake with my shipment. What? Oh, well, I got bags labeled 'One Meal' that are 1.13 ounces. That's right, one ounce. You know I'm a fat person, right?"

Eating them slow... hoping for strength...

April 29: Ugh. Day 2.

Complaints: headache, the oatmeal (gag! I only choked it down because I have no self-respect about food), not sleeping at all well last night.

Good things: the bars, shakes and eggs are all edible to me so far. Cottage cheese for breakfast was the yum. Scale showed a 2 pound drop this morning, which I know means nothing, but was still quite nice to see.

So far the complaints are outweighing the goodness in my mood, but it's just because I hate being headachy and tired. Well, who doesn't? Making some green tea and taking Alleve now...

April 30: Day 3. OMG Yeah, baby!

I feel amazing. Part of that is that we had a little family intervention last night so I'm off the hook for that particular bit of family drama for a little while—huge psychic energy wrapped up in it, and it's behind me now. And part of it is that my body is groovin' on this. I feel light, alert, sassy, satisfied by MF meals, and good to go! Just don't take away my Tony Chachere's. I'll put a hurtin' on you.

I am going to need to totally switch up my order for next time, and pray for MF to come out with more savory options. What is with all this sugary crap??!??! I know it's artificially sweetened, but I don't have that much of a sweet tooth. Once a day is MORE than enough for anything in the shake/bar/oatmeal/pudding/drink category. Sugar sugar sugar gack!

Today was awesome so far b/c I had MF eggs for breakfast and Chicken and Wild Rice soup for lunch, both of which I quite like, because they're *savory*. It's sweet bars and shakes from now until LG [LG or L&G is "Lean and Green," a meal of lean protein and low-carb vegetables, eaten once a day], which is not so great, but, well... next time. Maybe I'll place my order early for a bunch of savory stuff and spread out the shakes/puddings/nonsense over the next couple months.

I love my "before" pics. That super-fat chins and little fat-enveloped eyes profile picture hovers before my inner vision anytime I contemplate off-plan foods. No thank you—I can't believe I look like this, and it has to stop!

Hope everyone else is having a wonderful day too. Be well, stay OP!

April 30: Day 3. Strawberry Shake

It just took me *one entire hour* to eat the strawberry shake I had frozen. I kept forgetting about it.
Forgetting about it.
I had to make myself finish it. Now I am stuffed. Uh, *win*!

2 MAY

May 1: Started Wed. Day 4. Lost 5 pounds.

Okay, wow. I'm not even dehydrated. This is pretty neat. Let's see, at this rate, I'll be at goal in... five minutes. Just kidding—I'm not going there! I know this is for the long haul. But still, nice that the body responds so quickly with positive feedback.

Dinner last night was a revelation. It was the first time I tried to have my L&G all at once. A twenty-ounce package of 99% fat free ground turkey produces exactly two seven-ounce cooked portions. I had it with one and a half cups of cooked mushrooms. I use these salad plates usually for my food, and I could barely pile it all on there. No way was I going to be able to eat it at one sitting. I had to reheat the other half at 10:00 in order to finish. Needless to say it made me feel really good and safe to be able to fill my belly so satisfyingly at the end of the day.

I'm not sleeping well since I started. My body is all *waaahhhhooooo* and doesn't want to quiet down. Last night I took half a sleeping pill just so I could stabilize a little—my first law school exam of the semester is this Wed, and I need to start studying!

Yesterday I went to a reception for the dean of our school. It had the tables piled high with all the tasty tidbits—tarts, puffs, truffles, deep fried things, mini albacore sandwiches... I stood away from the tables and did not go stand within reach of them during the entire reception. I eyeballed them from across the room a lot, the way you eyeball your friend's hot new boyfriend, knowing you can't have it and trying not to get caught looking. When I was leaving I spotted celery and grabbed a handful. Chewing is good.

Today is my first restaurant challenge. I had organized dim sum with a dozen people—had set the date long before I decided to do MF. At this restaurant, they serve a steamed greens dish with a brown sauce that's drizzled—I should be able to scrape most of it off and have that for green. I can order "shrimp stuffed tofu" off the menu, which is pretty much just that. It's steamed also. I suspect there's some corn starch holding the shrimp together on top of the pieces of tofu, but I don't think it'll be too terribly off plan. So I figure I can avoid the tidbits, eat a dish I know I like, and stay OP. Wish me luck.

Five pounds!

May 2: Day 4.5. Can't sleep.

Anyone else have the onset of ketosis bring with it insomnia? I haven't been sleeping well since I started. Otherwise, I'm fine and doing well, but this is driving me a little batty.

I'm not sure that it helps that I'm lying in bed counting ounces of tofu and deciding what veggies I'll mix with my eggs tomorrow and and and... Obsess much? Noooooo....

May 2: Honestly? I'm busy saving my life.

As a starting point, being fat isn't that great for my health. While I don't have problems with my blood pressure, diabetes, etc, they'd be along eventually I'm sure. I do already have difficulty with physical exertion that other people would find minor, aching joints, back pain, I need custom ($500!) orthopedic inserts in my shoes to stave off the plantar fasciitis and walking fractures, etc.

I'm finishing up my 2nd year of law school. I started MF during *study days* before exams. On the one hand, this is pure idiocy because it's a lot to focus on, a huge change for my body, tiring, and incredibly distracting. On the other hand, it's not like I was doing that well before I started either.

(TMI ahead—move along, or proceed at your own risk)

I went to Mexico in early Feb for a week. I got cyanobacter, which is a lovely little organism that kills 1/1000 people infected. It gave me horrible bloody diarrhea—4 separate multi-day bouts. One morning I filled the bowl with blood and went to the emergency room for the first time since 1988. In the middle of that, I caught a cold and had pre-pneumonia, bronchial spasms for which my doc gave me an inhaler and codeine cough syrup, and used 4+ entire boxes of Kleenex in a week and a half. Sick sick sick... The diarrhea continued for an entire month—going to the bathroom 8–20 times a day. No one can live like that.

So I started gradually healing from that, where I was down to less than five BM/day, in mid-March. My body still doesn't want lettuce or other especially high-fiber vegetables. And I've remained spacey and had difficulty concentrating.

At this point I don't know who's doing what. How much is weight, stress, malabsorption of nutrients, torn-up gut, exhaustion, depleted immune system, mercury poisoning (j/k!), etc... I feel like the MF plan is giving me a chance to rest my gut some more. It's a lower volume of food, and most of it highly processed which makes for easy digestion. I'm starting with the more easily digestible veggies—mushrooms, hearts of palm, spaghetti squash...

I'm studying very slowly. I'm easily distracted, mostly by the MF boards. My first exam is Wed, and I have a Law Review mass edit I have to take care of tomorrow after work. Oh yeah, I have a full time job and go to school at night. But I still feel it was the right thing to start when I did. While the overachiever perfect student part of me is losing her mind at my unpreparedness, another part of me knows that the time was NOW.

I need to hang onto the big picture. My grade in the 2 classes I have exams in this term won't change the course of my life one way or another. Doing this amazing thing for my health will.

I'm an Aries, independent as hell, loathe to ask for help or admit vulnerability. But I admit it. My body is not okay. It's affecting my brain. And MF is the tool I choose today to turn that around.

May 3: got lab results

I had my doc do some of the basic hormone and lipid checks, just to rule out a medical issue. Everything was fine but my Vit D (low) and my cholesterol—high for the first time ever.

So, good timing for me! Time to turn that around and give my doc nothing to bitch about on my next visit. And phew! on the overall blood sugar/hormone front—nice to get the "all clear."

I am hungry today—I have a hard time with the sweet things being a meal. They just all leave me hungry. Think I'll walk to the store for some pickles and a break from my desk.

May 4: Is this even possible?

It's Day 7, not even a full week over yet, and I've lost an inch everywhere and 2 off my thighs. 6 pounds, too. But seriously, did I just forget how to use my tape measure between a week ago and today? REALLY?

May 5: Week one complete—7 pounds

That's it, really. Now, off to my Business Entities exam in... 7.5 hours and counting—ack!

May 6: Day 9: feeling fantastic

It doesn't hurt that my big scary Business Entities exam is over, and just the piddly crap I don't care about remains. But I think it's more than that—my body feels *sassy*!

Coworker sabotaged my legal career by bringing germs into work—fighting off the nasties. Which leads to an important question: do I count Dayquil as a condiment?

Total victory was mine yesterday. Exam day. Huge exam. Exam from 6:30–9:30 at night. Not feeling prepared, very stressed, slightly sick, hopped up on green tea and Dayquil. I stayed OP! My normal exam routine involves lots of extra protein and comfort foods. Yesterday I had turkey as my lean, because the 7 ounces makes me feel really full, and I had half of it around 1 and the other half at 6 just before the exam. I ate a bar during the exam. When I got home, all wired from the test, I did not eat more food I wasn't allowed. I had dill pickles, chicken broth, and cream cheese (I'd forgotten my healthy fats earlier). If I can stay OP on exam day, well, I think I can accomplish just about anything.

May 6: How to not be a fat person by the time I'm thin

I've been thinking about "fat people" and "thin people" and it's not all in the weight. I know someone who had one of those surgeries (not sure if it was the gastric bypass or the lap band) and has lost a TON of weight. But when he gets food, although he eats smaller portions he makes very high-fat choices. Someone else's friend had the surgery and kept drinking buckets of gravy. They are still fat people within, regardless of how their outsides looked. I log my food, obsess about when I get to eat next and what I'm going to eat, read the posts about food in the discussion groups, fantasize about new recipes to try, feel "safe" when I fill my belly with my L&G, etc.

But when I'm at my goal weight, I don't want to be a thin outside with a fat girl inside bursting at the seams to get out. I need to change that girl, change my thinking... I need to become someone who *wants* to make healthy eating choices, does it more naturally, and doesn't obsess so darn much about food.

Things are easing up slightly from the first few days. But I don't want to get complacent and not make the inner changes to go with the outer.

What have those who have maintained for a while changed in themselves? Are they just relentlessly vigilant? Have they reprogrammed things so it feels more natural? What can I do now, to change the fat girl within while I change the fat girl without?

May 10: Random cranky ranting

I have so much crabby in my pants today! I feel like tearing the heads off of small furry things, or coworkers, or customers— whichever talks to me first. ZOMG!

It's not TOM [Time of the Month] for another 8–12 days, so I don't think I can blame pre-menstrual. I've been getting plenty of sleep. I'm drinking my water, eating my healthy fats & all my MF meals & my full L&G.

Perhaps it's that I have an exam tomorrow for which I am epically unprepared. Epically. It's a multiple-choice exam, and his questions make no sense to me even when I have read the cases (which I haven't) or listened in class (which I haven't), so it's not like I had any sense of control anyway. I mean, what kind of a jackass tests ConLaw with a Scantron sheet? It's shameful. I am full of resentment to have to spend the next 32 hours with this class on my mind.

Also, I'm just pure evil. I never get this cranky! Anyone else hit a wall of crank-dom towards the end of week 2? Is this normal? *Roooorrrrwwwwwrrrr!*

(In other news, I've been 100% OP since the first couple days, I've lost 9 pounds and 2 inches off my waist, when I look down while walking I just see boobs and not belly, and my size 22 pants now can be pulled straight down without unzipping. But all that means nothing in the face of the *epic crankipants I am wearing*.)

May 10: so maybe we're not supposed to be happy all the time

I mean, really, *duh*, of course. But some lovely commenter (sorry, don't have that blog post open and forget who) said something about learning new ways to deal with our feelings that got me thinking.

What if we're just supposed to have crappy emotions sometimes? And NOT self-medicate them with food? It's not like losing weight or even being slender is going to magically make my life perfect and the world perfect and remove all hormonal fluctuations from my life.

So okay, sure, I need to learn new ways to deal with my emotions without food, in the middle of my crazy demented stressful fulltimework/lawschool life. But what if one of the coping mechanisms is to not even try to fix a crappy mood/day? Okay, I feel like crap today. I'm fussy. All day. And it might be because I'm a little sick, it might be because of exams, it might be because I haven't been laid in a century or two, it might because the moon is in the second dogstar of Aquarius trined my butt, it might be because my body is *freaking out* with all these MF changes, it might be because I'm hungry, might might might. I could run around and try to remove all the stressors. I could go get therapy. I could eat.

Or, I could just sit in the crabby and see what tomorrow brings. I think I'd like to try that today.

May 11: And a new day dawns....

I'm in a great mood today. 2 weeks, 11 pounds, 3 inches off my waist. *ZOMG!*

Please people, just slap me if I ever start talking about how "easy" this diet is—I know that amnesia will kick in at some point. Just remind me that I had to drug myself to sleep the first week so I didn't lie there obsessing about what I got to eat when and how much I wanted to be eating it now, and all the other teensy little moment-to-moment challenges. But so worth it!

11 pounds. That ain't all water weight, bee-atches! I am hoping that within a month I'll start hearing that people besides me can tell.

Have a fantastic day!

May 12: Mood Swings of DOOM—Week 3

I'm about ready to put myself on an emotional "time out." You know when you know you're PMSing, so you don't really believe you're as upset as you feel you are—you discount it somewhat because you know you're hormonal? Same thing if you're really tired, or getting sick...

Well, my moods are sproinking up and down like little cute bunnies, and then they turn into slimy toads, and somewhere in here I lost track of my metaphor but the point is *"Sheesh!* I'm giving women a bad name!"

Crabby, giddy, despairing, calmly confident, exhausted, relaxed, full of energy—and that's just the highlights from the past 3 days. I'm giving myself whiplash.

Today started all "oh, poor me, this is really hard, someone tell me I can do this" and has transitioned into "I've totally got this, this is awesome, I'm just fine, I can't wait to go buy a Starbucks cup after work." I'm like a four-year-old. A very annoying one.

May 13: Last night I dreamed...

...that I could cross my legs. This tells me my "visioning" is sinking itself into my subconscious. I'm a bit startled to see myself in the mirror now—not in the "cringe" way, but in the "oh, we aren't quite there yet? Well, I love watching you shrink, girl!" kind of way.

I've been spending so much time seeing myself in this little pink dress with neutral stockings and these completely adorable Steve Madden shoes in my closet from a couple springs ago that I've never worn—they're high high heels in Easter pastel colors—turquoise, pink, and yellow. With a pink dress, I shall be so freakin' adorable total strangers will fall to their knees and beg to take a bite out of my ass.

You gotta have a vision, right?

May 14: going to 4&2

I've been having a conversation with the dietitians on the boards about whether I should be doing 5&1 or 4&2. I'm switching to 4&2. [5&1 is 5 Medifast meals and 1 Lean and Green meal a day. 4&2 is 4 Medifast meals and 2 Lean and Green meals a day. 4&2 has a couple hundred more calories a day, but still stays below 1200 per day.]

Emotionally, I am all frickin' conflicted about this. On the one hand, I feel all like I failed at the 5&1 and I have this guilty thing that makes me keep feeling like I have to justify myself. SO, here is the official justification, and I'm going to put it on paper like I were defending myself in court, and try to get that guilty weasely whiner to STFU:

1) The dietitian recommended I do it.
2) It is recommended for people with 50+ pounds to lose to start with more food, as you need more energy.
3) The dietitian said that it can help prevent early plateaus.
4) The dietitian said it's recommended if your energy is low or if you're experiencing daily hunger.
5) I am hungry every day.
6) I am not craving junk, and it doesn't seem to be emotionally triggered. What I want is 99% ff ground turkey, scallops,

etc—things high in protein and low in fat. Which makes me think my body is just really needing more fuel.
7) My energy levels are most definitely low. Also really erratic. If this can help smooth them out I'm all for it.

So, I am going to try to go with the attitude that I know I *can* do the 5&1, as I did it for 2.2 weeks. But I'm *choosing* to go with the recommendation and what I think is the wisdom of my body (and not the inner junkie). I'm going to try 4&2 and see how it goes, and if all goes well, when I get to Onederland [under 200 pounds] I'll switch back to 5&1.

I'm not going all the way to the diabetic 4-2-1 thing, because I just don't see the point of adding carbs back in with the extra "healthy snack"—I'm already through withdrawal.

Phew. It's such a mess inside my head.

May 15: Oh what a difference a couple hundred calories makes

Now I know 4&2 isn't for everybody. I'm doing it because the dietitian recommended it for people with more than 50 pounds to lose. And while I know it will slow my weight loss some, it turns out to only increase my day's total calorie intake by a couple hundred, and my carbs remain below 100.

And I feel completely different. The body-panic feeling vanished from one day to the next. It's not like I suddenly get to indulge every phantom craving—it's still 1135–1245 calories/day (so far). But the extra protein is making all the difference for my hunger and making me feel good in my body about the diet.

I finally feel like I get to *enjoy* the ketosis! I'm so glad I listened to that advice...

Oh, and I'm down 2 more pounds. 13 now!

May 18: It's hard to feel too deprived...

... when my mid-morning snack is comprised of fresh cherry tomatoes and crab dip (crab, ricotta, garlic, and Worcestershire sauce). Um, yeah. Totally suffering.

14 pounds down and hitching up my pants all the time. Loving it.

Last night I had a little personal victory. I had eaten my snack a little early, and stayed up a little late, and I was a teensy bit hungry when I went to bed. I have always been really bothered by the feeling of going to bed hungry. Last night I just told myself I was out of food for the day and there was nothing more to eat. I embraced the feeling instead of fighting it. And I did go to sleep, instead of lying awake fretting about it. Okay, this feels kind of major for me.

May 19: Starting Week 4—wow!

3 full weeks down, 14 pounds, 3.5 inches off my waist. Amazing. I am one pound from my first mini-goal.

Last night I had another new experience—the first time it was hard to eat all my food. I had half my dinner L&G at 6, and would normally eat the other half at 8—I'm on an every-other-hour schedule for meals. But I didn't eat it until 8:45 because I just didn't want it, and then it was hard to get through.

This is kind of spectacularly wonderful. It's not to say I wouldn't have eaten several other things if I could eat whatever I wanted again. I am feeling the lack of "food as entertainment" the last couple days. But the vision I have of myself thinner is currently worth far more to me than some ephemeral oral pleasures.

I also want to say that if they take cream cheese off the list of approved healthy fats, I will never ever recognize it. My denial will be utter and complete. OMG cream cheese. (I have a small voice inside that is starting to recognize that it's too heavy and filling, and in not very long I'll be using more flax seed oil and less cream cheese, but that little voice is for later and I'm not listening to it now nananananananayoucan'tmakemenananannanana *fingers in ears*.)

May 19: Anyone ever check out People of Walmart...

... to feel better about themselves? Turns out I am slim, lovely, and a paragon of fashion.

May 20: 14 pounds

Well, I was briefly beating myself up because I'm sitting around on my sofa watching TV for the second night in a row. (After just finishing my law school semester a week ago, and I work full time, and I did loads of housecleaning and cooking for 3 days before that. But all that has *nothing* to do with today's self-flagellation.)

Anyway, mental train of thought started like this: "Gosh there's so much to do around the house I really should be doing it." Then I looked down at the pile of bags of Epsom salts in the bathroom waiting for me to reorganize the closet so they'll all fit (I was stocking up. I do that with everything, now, since I never have time to shop while school's happening. There are big stacks of identical boxes all over my house, it's hilarious. Find the bathroom cabinet where I store the Emergen-C, and lo and behold there are 6 boxes! Locate the extra hand soap? 4 giant jugs of it. Tuna? *Two* Costco packages of it. Who needs *two* Costco size anythings? Oh, and don't get me started on the apocalypse-sized stores of cat food.)

I pick up three full four-pound bags of Epsom salts. And a half-full bag. And I have 14 pounds in my arms. It's heavy. It's unwieldy, and they slip around a little. It's definitely annoying. I dance around with it for a minute, just to see what I was carrying with every step, every breath, just 3 weeks ago, that is now gone forever.

14 pounds. And I'm going to do that, what, 5 more times? 85 pounds (my goal loss) is 21 large four-pound bags of Epsom salts. I can't fit that many in my bathroom, much less in my arms.

So, the housecleaning can wait. The amount of energy I'll have for it in a few more weeks will be so much more than now, the more giant sacks of fat I set down and don't pick up again. I'm a little misty thinking about it, and I am starting to get why people totally burst into tears in dressing rooms.

I am so grateful to have this program and all this support. This is a wonderful community and it's an honor to be here.

Now if you'll excuse me, I have some cream cheese to eat. Yay, healthy fats! *grin*

May 21: Keeping a close eye on my boobs

... and belly. I'm waiting for the day when my belly no longer sticks out farther than my boobs. Yes, I am an apple-shaped girl!

I figure my belly needs to shrink another inch or two. Well, or boobs need to grow (ha!). Maybe another 10 pounds? Can't wait. Every time I go into the bathroom I turn sideways and check. I think I'm going to need to rig up a plumb bob to dangle over my shoulder for a scientific determination. When it hangs free off the ta-tas, we're officially there.

I no longer unzip my pants to take them on and off. I have a feeling these 22s are not going to last too much longer. And this morning I met my first mini-goal of 220, 15 pounds down.

May 24: how am I doing?

Well, let's see:

1) MediGassy. *ZOMG!* I took a break from bars today, and still—wow! Impressive gurgling sounds from within.
2) Lonely and sad and fussy and crabby and hating everyone and short-tempered and unwilling to be at work and totally unproductive. *I miss overeating and stuffing my feelings very much thank you.* I can haz KFC nao?
3) In the groove with the MF. Liking it. Boring myself with the egg beaters and ground turkey, but hey—it's been really good to be so full. Having a hard time eating it all. (Yay!) I'll change up my lean next Costco trip—in the meantime, repetition is the price of volume discounts, for those who dine alone.
4) Feeling very betwixt and between. I've lost a giant pile of lard off myself—16 pounds is 21 of those 12-ounce packages of bacon. That's a lot. But I'm still 219 pounds on a 5'2" frame and a long way to go before goal.
5) More energy is nice. Very nice. My house is getting cleaner. I'm doing more things, walking more.
6) Waiting for my big reveal. I have some things I'm actively not doing now, while I focus on this project. Partly because one huge project is enough. Partly because, well, how can I

shop for men when I'm changing my body so drastically? It's just false advertising to date now. Finding a guy who digs me like this can certainly be accomplished if I feel I'm good and over the ex (status pending on that determination), but what's the point? I'll be a totally different chick in a few months. I've never been one to delay anything because I'm a BBW, so this is kind of a strange mindset, but even though I feel lonely I also feel like hermitting up and really concentrating on this project until I get a bit further along.

7) School starts in one week. I'm not sure there are enough hours in the day for all the TV I want to watch before that happens.

May 25: Wow. Today blows.

I feel overwhelmed at work, and people have apparently designated today as "Be An Aggressive Hostile Prick For No Reason and Yell at Freya" Day. As if we needed one of those. To celebrate the day, people are calling and yelling from as far away as Belgium. Now that's special.

Which situation is not helped by all the free-floating anxiety and hostility I have, because *I cannot overeat to comfort myself* and I am very *angry* about this. (Said in Pretty Woman voice: "I am very *angry* with my father.")

I had to register for Beverage Law of all absurd things because I'm waitlisted for two other classes I actually want to take in that time slot.

Also, did I mention I can't overeat to deal with this? WTF? I am so not okay with today. Good thing I can leave work in 2 hours and confine myself to my quarters.

And yet, it's an *OP day*!

PS: why do I not have a post tag category below for "Rage and Hostility"? Don't they know we're fat people on *diets*? Where's the compassion?

May 28: Single girl loves the weekends

I keep seeing people all stressed out about the holiday weekend and how hard it will be to stay OP. And I just want to say this is one case where being a grumpy misanthropic antisocial single law student *really* comes in handy.

I will be bunkered in most if not all of the weekend. I have food, I don't have any plans after tonight, and all I really need to do is read for the first week of one class (starts Tuesday ack!) and cook some L&G for next week. I might putter on house projects/cleaning. I will definitely watch a lot of TV. I will take bubble baths.

And best of all, I will sleep in, and go to bed early. MF has made it so I'm actually tired at night! I go to bed between 9:30 and 10:30 every night now, without even trying. And on the weekends, I can wake up at my usual time, stretch, pee, and go back to sleep for 4 more hours of recreational bliss.

Then, when I finally haul my ass out of bed, I've missed two regularly scheduled mealtimes. In order to get all my food in, I feel like I'm pretty much eating all day. Which makes me really happy.

I know it sounds like I'm a total depressive, but I work full time and do law school at night, and somewhere along the way I lost my "guilt setting" for the unabashed sloth I engage in during term breaks. When I'm in school, a "study break" looks an awful lot like "dishes" or "laundry" and I'm happy for it because at least I'm not reading about stock options or federal regulations. So anyway, yay! A long weekend of sloth. Interrupted by whatever movement and productivity my shrinking bod feels like doing, with no pressure from me whatsoever.

And no pressure or temptation from the world about what I eat. *happy sigh*

May 28: Not ready for prime time

I'm an emotional eater going through serious crazy messed-up withdrawal from my favorite form of comfort. I am meeting people for dinner tonight. And I don't feel ready for the challenges of ordering off a menu, negotiating fat content with the waiter at a very busy restaurant, estimating volumes/weights, filling in at home, etc. I'm just going to have some tea. However rude that makes me, I'm just having tea. I'll eat before and after, at home, with my weighed and measured food.

I am feeling very proud of myself for recognizing that I'm not ready to improvise yet. I will be, soon enough. But not while I'm still yelling in the car as I drive past Burgermaster about how everything would feel so much better if I could just have a cheeseburger and onion rings. When spontaneous swearing at fast food places is a regular experience, I'm not ready to take off the training wheels.

And that's just fine. I'm still OP, I'm down 17 pounds in 4 weeks, and aside from the terrible vile mood swings I feel pretty darn good.

May 31: Starting to get a sense of peace—5 weeks in

I'm getting to where I can almost relax about this. Really simple plain foods taste fantastic, but I don't much care if they don't. I'll eat them anyway. It's fuel. Today's strawberry shake cake was halfway to vile, and I just didn't really give a rat's patooty. I've been having some shrimp for my lean, and here's my high-tech recipe: 7 oz cooked shrimp from Costco, dumped in a bowl with 1 T Newman's light Italian, with a sprinkling of salt. Yeah. Fancy.

My other lean this week is a truly fine cut of beef, broiled, with baked mushrooms and bell peppers. Nothing heavily flavored. I'm eating my cabbage plain with some salt.

I used to be all foodie up in here, but not anymore! Now my taste buds are digging on the simple flavors. If I put hot sauce on something, my stomach rebels a little.

I like the schedule, a lot. I know what I get to eat, when. I know I won't die on this diet. My body is trusting that I won't starve to death. The 4&2 is working really well for me. I put the MF crackers and soy crisps back on the "only in case of emergency" list, because they felt like a little too much carbs, and a leeetle too delicious.

I did go off plan a teensy bit yesterday. I grilled the filet. I was slicing it. I was not planning to have filet yesterday for my lean, I had another meal already cooked that needed to be eaten. But hot, tender, melt-off-the-fork steak won, and I ate about an ounce. Well, if I have to have a trigger that makes me go off plan, steak isn't the worst one. Count it and move on!

Hope everyone is having a lovely end to the long weekend.

3 JUNE

June 1: Fear

I've identified another fear to be cataloged and then moved past. I am afraid that when I remove the weight I'll uncover a woman who's not that pretty anymore and just plain old. I haven't been at my goal weight since I was 26–27, and I'm 41 now.

When I look at people's after pics, sometimes I think they look better. Sometimes I think they look worse—pinched, chicken-necked, old, without the softness and grace that some extra padding can give you.

So, here I go into the unknown, not at all sure who will look back out of the mirror at me when I'm done. For sure this ain't time travel, and it won't be that fresh pretty 26-year-old girl. I hope I like the new person who I uncover.

But, I'm trying to tell myself that worst case—I was "conventionally unattractive" fat, and even if I'm "conventionally unattractive" thin, it'll be a healthy thin that wears clothes well. So it has to be a net benefit.

I just hope I like my new face.

June 2: Mood Swing UP!

Ya'all have been getting such an earful of the mood swings down I thought I'd share the other side. I've had a couple weeks of feeling like I was careening around inside one of those triangle things you use for setting up pool balls—with the corners labeled "rage" "loneliness" and "sadness." But last night I was on the phone with my best girl, who is going through a horrible breakup. She was in a pretty good space, but not quite good enough to explain why she kept giving me the giggles. I couldn't stop laughing. I finally said "I don't know what's wrong with me, I feel a little drunk!"

She said "you're clearly malnourished and overwrought." And I laughed a lot more.

June 4: What kind of f'ing idiot picks a diet that doesn't allow bingeing?

Me. That's what kind.

I hear that WW lets you game the points so you can still binge on your favorite foods. South Beach lets you eat all you want of certain veggies. And Atkins—well, you can pretty much sit down and tuck into a tub of lard whenever you want.

But MF? No, not MF. Those rotten devious evil rat bastids have designed a program that is so regimented in every area that there's not a single teensy thing that one can eat and eat and eat until one feels better.

"One," of course, being "me."

I was never a girl who would eat a dozen doughnuts, or a puker. I have always been able to eat part of a bag of chips. I generally ate 5 small meals a day. But when I needed comfort, I could eat a can of chili with cream cheese in it (or a plate of fried pot stickers or whatever fatty protein-rich equivalent caught my eye) and get *full*. Full enough to feel *better*. That's what tells me I'm a food addict. That it would make me feel better and without it I'm bereft.

I've been having all the mood swings as the feelings I can no longer stuff come up. Last night, the grief hit. I was watching Benjamin Bratt's *The Cleaner*, and I realized that I can *never* eat that way again. The same way an alcoholic has to let go of the idea of ever drinking again. (I'm not saying that in 5 or 10 years I couldn't go wild at dim sum on occasion, after getting very solid in my sobriety as to the emotional component of my eating, but I am saying that for a very long *now* I need to just *stop* so I can unhook the emotional associations with food.)

I had a cry. A whiny pathetic pity party cry, grieving the loss of the idea of that comfort. The loss of the reality of that comfort. Surrendering to knowing that I cannot have that particular good feeling any more. I cried about how hungry I am and how tired I am of being hungry. I didn't want to eat, though. I was just very sorry for myself and sad and went to bed hungry and didn't lie there thinking about things I could eat. I just laid there and cried about how bad I felt.

It blows. Boy did I pick the right diet.

June 7: It's unwinding somewhat...

The longer I stay OP, the more the deep freaked-out food-issue parts of me recognize some new truths:

1) It doesn't matter how much they whine, scream, cry, pout, and/or rage, even all at once—they don't get more food.
2) I don't die. Not even a little.
3) Hunger is not an emergency. And I can pretty much always live through 2 hours until my next meal.

I found myself doing some exciting revolutionary things this weekend:

1) I chose L&Gs that came in smaller portions, and without extra healthy fats [when you choose extremely lean meats/fish, you supplement them with healthy fats], because they were what I was in the mood to eat. I knew I'd be fuller with some egg beaters in my day, but I also knew that my hunger wouldn't kill me so who cares?
2) I stayed up late. Not really late, but 11:00. I've been going to bed by 10 for a couple/few weeks—just really tired at 9:45 and off to bed I go. Last night I wasn't tired so I watched another episode and went to bed at 11. This is revolutionary and exciting because I'd had my last food for the day before 9:00. Last week I would have been scared to be awake still when I got hungry again. Last night, I didn't care if I went to bed hungry when I did go to bed—I knew I'd still be able to sleep.

I'm not going to say anything crazy like "I didn't think about food all day" or anything. Because I did. But it's getting better, and last week's crushing grief isn't here now, and for all of that I'm very grateful.

Oh, and best of all, after a week with no movement on the scale, I dropped 3 pounds over the weekend. I'm officially 25% of the way to goal, in just under 6 weeks. W00t!

June 8: I thought I had a little more time…

… before this particular feeling appeared. This morning I went from 22s to 20s. Now, I know the 22s were starting to look ridiculous, like I'd had a continence issue of the second kind. But they were the pants I was comfortable in. Nice and baggy and loose.

The 20s, they actually fit. They're actually more comfortable, because they're not shifting around all over the place and having to be hitched up. But I have that feeling: the insecure exposed feeling. I thought for sure I'd have more time before that appeared. *sigh* Well, we'll start dealing with it now!

I also made a Leaning Tower of Pants. I fished out all the smaller sized pants from my closet, and sorted them by size. I have about a week's worth of pants each in 20, 18, and 16. After that… it's the Goodwill Lending Library. And time travel. Below 16 is a Long Long and Scary Time Ago, Before All the Bad Breakups.

I guess I'll deal with all the horrors of being that little when I get there. No point in borrowing that trouble today. Today I have to deal with the anxieties of being *this* little. *grin*

Now, before people jump all over the helpful suggestions—this isn't actually any sort of problem that needs fixing. This is a *feeling* which I need to acknowledge and work through so it doesn't make me sabotage myself later.

June 11: on second thought, I leapfrogged the 20s

I wore them for 2 days. And then I admitted that they were also baggy and ridiculous. I set aside the rest of the stack of 20s and started in on the 18s. *happy sigh* Now that's how a pair of jeans are supposed to fit.

June 12: It's pretty much been made of awesome around here lately...

Let me enumerate:

1) The aforementioned 18s. Bye-bye to 24, 22, and 20. Seeya! Go right ahead and let the door hitcha, I don't give a rat's ass.
2) More and more energy. Also sparkle. Boys are starting to notice. Like wanting to hang out and talk a little longer than is reasonable.
3) A boy showed off. No, really! A twenty-ish boy was crossing the street in front of my car, and he caught my eye. I gave him a little half smile. I was in a really good mood. When he got to the curb, he leapt in the air and spun around on his way back down to the ground. Then he caught my eye again, just to make sure I'd seen. *So adorable!* I haven't had a boy show off for me in so long. It's good to have my sparkle coming back.
4) Food: it's made of deliciousness. Today's salad—spring greens, fresh tomatoes, the pre-cooked plain grilled chicken from Costco. I contemplated salad dressing. I thought, "I don't want to waste a fat on that." I tried it without dressing. *Yum!* Best salad I've ever eaten. A little salt, that was it. So freaking good—all the flavors in the greens.... Wow. Taste buds change much?
5) Food: bad food is made of gross. I had a very strong experience the other day driving home, when I thought about McDonalds and was physically nauseous. Then I tried KFC, same result. My body was completely, 100% sure it did not want any of that anywhere near it. Toxins clearing out! This episode involved a lot of hysterical laughter and screaming, because once I started thinking of foods that made me ill, and then tried to *stop* thinking of them, well, it's like saying "don't think about pink elephants." It was all I could think of. I was laughing so hard my stomach hurt.

6) Food: today it became very clear I'm eating too much food. This week I had ground turkey with some egg beaters as my lean, and it was just too much. I'm shifting to salads with salmon and chicken this week, to lighten things up. I'm a little shocked that I have a body that is now willing to say "yeah, I know it's less than 1200 calories a day and all (I'm still on 4&2), but it's too much." Who am I?
7) I'm shopping for bodies. Walking around Costco, I'm checking all the women out. "That one? No, a little too skinny. How about that one? I like the amount of junk in that trunk. Do I want to be all muscular like that one?" Seriously. It's like window-shopping. For my new body.

June 12: Eeek! Wish me luck!

First time eating someone else's food since I started MF! I'm spontaneously driving to Portland to see my cousin (3 hours 22 minutes according to Mapquest) and driving back again after hanging out for a couple hours. His family is moving to California, and I thought they were leaving the end of the month but I just found out this weekend is my last chance to see them before they go.

Wheee—to the batmobile!

Anyway, I'm like "we don't have to eat or anything, we can just hang out," and he's all "We'll grill!" Okay, cool. He asks about dietary restrictions, I'm like "I'm pretty much just eating meat/seafood and veggies, so anything on the grill and a salad would be awesome." So.... here I go.... letting go of control. I plan to not freak out if there is grated carrot in the salad or if it's already dressed. I want to just go have a semi-normal dinner with family, and I'll do the best I can to leave what's off plan on the plate.

But I'm kind of thrilled to have a new diet adventure. I've only eaten food I've prepared since 4/28. Entirely. No restaurants, no takeout, no family meals, no dinner at friends' houses, no nothing. I've been in the bunker where it's safe.

Here I go, leaving the bunker. I feel ready. I'm totally excited to spread my wings a little, and let my new tools/mind/body/awareness support me in a new food environment that's not so rigidly "safe" for me.

And, *eeek!*

June 13: Dinner with family—first time out of the bunker. And first *roadtrip!*

Who doesn't snack all day when driving a long distance (7.5 hours driving total yesterday)? I *always* used food to keep me alert and entertained in the car. If I was eating healthy, it was kumquats—they take a while to eat and are tart/sweet/seeds entertainment for your mouth. If not eating healthy... well, you know.

I did *great!* In the car, I ate on schedule. I had bars and puffs and started the drive with a shake. When I got there, we took the kids and dogs to the park and I slipped a bar into my back pocket and took a water bottle, because I needed to eat in 30 minutes and my spidey-senses told me we wouldn't be back from walking dogs and eating in half an hour. I ate my bar and when we had dinner an hour and a half later I wasn't too hungry.

They were really sweet and asked me what I would eat before they made things, and I helped with the salad. They cooked prawns on the grill instead of in a pan with butter, since that was how I would eat them. Also filet mignon. Yum! I asked for a small steak, and no, I couldn't weigh it. Since they had cooked the shrimp plain (not like it wasn't an option they were considering anyway, it was, but they chose that from among other options for me), I took two of those. So I had an unweighed piece of meat that might have been anywhere from 5–7 ounces and 2 shrimp. I had salad that was lettuce, cukes, radishes, and bell peppers, with no dressing. I won't bother to list the 800 different delicious tempting junk food things they ate in front of me. Like Doritos with creamy cheese and salsa, and fresh strawberries. But *nay nay*, I was *strong*.

I'm counting that as an OP meal, and a total success. The ride back home was a little stressful as there was a stretch of road south of Tacoma where they narrowed a 4-lane freeway down to 1. It took 50 minutes to go 5 miles, and I didn't get home until 11. I had an extra MF meal with me, but I didn't eat it. I waited until I got home and had the other half of my 2nd L&G (I'm on 4&2) as planned.

I did really good. It took a fair amount of negotiating, and of course they're all concerned that living on 1100 calories a day is really bad for me, but whatever. I was so glad I went. It was great to get to see them before they head off to the wilds of California. And I'm thrilled that I was so successful with an environment that is normally all about the junk food for me—*road trip!*

June 15: too gosh darned much food

The last week or so I've been feeling like I'm eating too much food. Seriously. 1100ish calories a day, and it's too much food (I'm on 4&2). Also, by splitting my 1st L&G I've been able to eat every 2 hours all day long. And that feels like too often.

Uh, who am I? Really? I'm feeling too full and a little icky on 1100 calories a day?

Yes, really.

I switched to salmon on green salads for my L&G, which drops me to 969 calories/day, and 70 grams carbs. Also, today I'm shifting my schedule to be eating every 2.5 hours pretty much. I've still got split L&Gs during the day, so I have as many meals to get in, but I moved one of my MF meals to "after dinner snack" so I can space the day out better. I'll have it instead of my dill pickle ritual. So I'm eliminating one time per day that I've been eating.

When I am ready to switch to 5&1, all I have to do is replace one of my L&G times with a MF meal, and I'll be good to go, and already on the right schedule. So far, so good. I ate at 10:30 instead of 10, and I'm eating in 20 minutes at 1 instead of at noon. And I'm not freaking out.

This is a really strange weaning process. But I feel fantastic. Yesterday I was like, "All I have to do is sit here. Here. I'm here, and all I have to do is Sit. Right. Here. and the weight will keep falling off." I'm not fighting an uphill battle against my cravings and my mind and emotions all day. What a relief.

I'm down 23 pounds, over 25% of the way to goal. 7 weeks in.

June 17: Today. Wow.

Totally freakin' insane with the hungries today, for like 4 hours this afternoon. And then I had to go to a catered reception, with tables of delicious savory pastries and fantasticness. My friend at law school who knows I'm on MF totally caught me leering at the carbs like a starving hyena. Luckily, my fellow students were bigger starving hyenas, and the table was pretty well cleared within about 15 minutes. But *boy howdy* was it hard to stay OP for a few minutes there.

Hungry day! Let's hope it shows up as a loss on tomorrow's scale...

June 18: Just whining. Don't even bother reading this.

I feel like dog turds today! I woke up with a little bit of a cough. I don't feel really sick, just slow and punky and bloated and tired. Puh. I can't wait to get home to a) my sofa or b) my tub, and either way there *will* be a TV involved.

There probably has to be a Costco stop on the way home, as going there on Sat/Sun makes me want to stab myself through the eye with a kabob skewer, but Fri night isn't too bad. And I just can't afford to buy my green anywhere else. This week I went through Costco-sized containers of lettuce, cucumbers, tomatoes, bell pepper, and *two* of mushrooms. 4&2 requires a lot of greens!

An hour and 40 minutes is the earliest I could take off from work without being a total jerk. 2 hours is better.

hanging on with slightly skinnier than before fingertips

June 19: One little crack in the wall of my shopping resolve

I wasn't going to do it. I wasn't going to buy *anything* until I was off the small end of everything I have in my closet. No clothes, no shoes, no nothing. No point, right? I can shop in my closet for now, and soon enough I'll be in the 16s and then they'll be falling of me and I'll *have* to shop.

But now, no shopping. That was the *rule*.

And then we went to DSW. Cuteness! So I bought one little pair. They have chunky heels, and the upper is all elastic so my feet feel super secure. I can wear them now, for things like out to dinner or something where I'm not walking a ton. And the more weight I drop, the longer I'll be able to wear them without my knees giving me an eviction notice.

So I have new cute shoes, that aren't 3–4+ years old from before I got so fat. And I'm kind of really excited about them.

June 22: Progress Update

I feel horrible today, emotionally, because I had way disturbing dreams last night. All about my food issues. Ick.

So, to make myself feel better, I'm focusing on my success so far:

- a week shy of 2 months
- 25 pounds gone forever
- 6 inches off my waist
- staying OP the whole time—no significant cheating
- down 3 sizes, from 24 to 18
- 30% of the way to goal.

That doesn't suck. Today does, but that does not.

June 23: Taking care of myself

After perfect attendance at my summer class so far, last night I played hooky. I left work a couple hours early ("I have an appointment. Yeah, now. That I didn't tell you about before, sorry.") I drove forthwith to the spa, and plunked my tookus down in some hot water. Also cold water, steam room, and sauna. I laid in a lawn chair and did some meditating, sorting through all my various stressors and current issues and deciding what I was going to do right now about each. (The overall consensus for most of them: nothing. But at least I feel better about it.)

Then I had a massage. Nice woman from North Carolina, so we reminisced about the South and made fun of women who breast feed too long and lamented the state of Seattle men, and other happy nonsense. Also a great massage.

Then I went home and watched TV and did not eat off plan. Pretty good day, for how stressed and tight I was earlier.

NSVs [Non-Scale Victories]: at the spa they give you a quick up-and-down when you walk in the door and they hand you the size robe they think you need. Last night's verdict: XL. For the first time in a loooooong time.

Today I went to put on a sparkly shirt I don't wear that often, and I was going to wear it "one last time" while big. Only it was a tent.

Actually unwearable. So I rummaged in the closet until I was late for work, and am now wearing an XL shirt I haven't worn in forever. It fits great. My pants are a little lose. I may totally love MF. Maybe. Just a little.

June 25: Visiting the place where they keep the food...

I needed to see my long-lost loves. On Monday it's 2 full months on MF, and, well, I needed to fondle fruit. Smell berries. Gasp at the wonder of a ripe nectarine. Eyeball ranch dressing, pastas, dried apricots, bright green pesto and olives, big jugs of oil, exotic spices, artichoke bruschetta spreads, shumai, brownie mix, corn meal, and lord only knows what else. I went up and down the aisles lingering lovingly, communing with all the foodie wonders of my favorite slightly upscale market.

What did I eat? Nothing. No sample cheeses found their way to my mouth. What did I buy? Cabbage, kim chi (I know, more cabbage), exotic salts (Real Salt, mined from prehistoric deposits, and pink Himalayan salt in large sexy crystals), jalapeno hot sauce, fresh salsa, garlic powder, and 3 flavors of Pam. If kim chee is not OP, please don't tell me for at least a week. I found one with no sugar or MSG and my mouth is in serious heaven right now.

It's a nice shift from *"don't look don't meet its eye or you'll die die die"* which is how I've been feeling about off plan foods for the last 2 months. I've been doing this covert lustful leer from afar when around them, but getting away as fast as I can. When I grocery shop, it's been these surgical strikes into Costco for like 5 items (3 veggies, a meat/fish, and dill pickles) and *out again before it gets me ZOMG!* But I felt no temptation whatsoever, just fond nostalgia and some gentle groping. Like seeing an ex-boyfriend you still like to cuddle up to but really don't want to sleep with. This felt like a good healthy place to be in my road to recovery, even if it was a bit batshit.

June 26: I ate out. First time.

My friend and I went shopping today, and she was holding me hostage. I had left home with my breakfast shake I was still working on, 2 bars and a bag of pretzels in my purse. I thought we'd be out for a couple hours because I wanted to pick up Just One Thing. *Ha!* But I've learned to be prepared with her, so I had food with me.

She held me hostage from 11am until 7pm. I finally just made my escape and back to home. So a couple awesome things—first, all the walking I did had to be good for me. Everything hurts so it must have been plenty of exercise. Ow my feet!

Then, I stocked up on good things for skin. I got like 10 tubs of body butter, some skin firming cream, Udderly Smooth lotion, and some bubble bath.

I got 2 belts! The 18W pants I'm wearing are starting to shift around annoyingly, and I'm small enough now to buy a normal-size-range belt at the thrift store. I got one that's perfect now on the biggest setting, so I can shrink into the other holes. Then, I got a smaller belt that'll be just perfect when I run out of holes on the larger one. It's the kind that has big grommety holes the whole length of it, so it can be any size. That should hold me until pretty much goal, and then I can get ones that will fit my new size once I know what it is.

I got a muffin pan for oatmeal muffins. I got new fry pans to replace the ones where the nonstick is wearing off—a small one for MF eggs, and a 9.5" for egg beaters. I got a couple more sets of measuring spoons at the dollar store, so I now have *four* tablespoons which I can lick cream cheese out of for my healthy fats.

I also did the *bad thing* that my mother always forbade—I bought clothes that don't fit me yet! I got a lovely black silk tank top—the knit kind of silk that's more like cashmere but is silk and drapes beautifully—it's a size large. I'm in XL–1X tops now, so I have to wait, but I have it to inspire me. And I got a medium shirt in a black slinky fabric that ZIPS all the way up the front, with ruching all along the sides of the zipper. It looks tough and sexy, but not whorish so I can even wear it to class if I'm going out after. It can hang on my bedroom door just looking good until I can fit in it.

Oh, it was a grand day for consumerism. All at the dollar store, Ross, TJ Max, and the thrift store—everything cheap and on sale and a big pile of loot in the entry way.

The best part of the day, though, was eating out at Outback Steakhouse. I had not had a single restaurant meal since April 27th, before I started MF. I wasn't planning to today. But my friend was hungry, and I did some quick mental calculations and reorganized my day, and I ordered food. A 6 ounce steak (can't be more than 4.5

cooked, so fine for lean), and my 2 sides were green beans and broccoli, steamed no butter. I sprinkled an indecent amount of salt on everything and it was so good! I was satisfied with my meal, and it didn't take 10 minutes of dickering with the waiter to order it. Super easy, and now I feel so much more confident about eating out.

All in all, *hooray!* What a good day.

June 27: OMG scallops.

That's really all I have to say. 7 ounces of scallops, pan-seared in 1/2 tsp of hot chinese oil. Eaten by themselves so I can really focus on their splendor.

Soon I shall follow them with kim chi. Eaten slowly while reading Evidence, as if it's a delicious snack food. Hooray!

June 28: I have an announcement

I was going to keep it to myself for a while, I think because I'm afraid of failing. *But*, I will not fail, because as Chris so eloquently said, I want this. I want it bad.

So, I'm switching from 4&2 back to 5&1. Today. My original plan was to wait to switch until Onederland, but for the last couple weeks I've often felt I'm eating too much food, or too often. I changed my eating schedule to every 2.5 hours instead of 2, and that made it much better. I'm watching my hunger cycle, and I get really *starved* in the 3:00 zone every day. So I'm having my one L&G during the lunch/early afternoon time, perhaps split, perhaps not. And just having MF for dinner.

This is mentally very scary to me. I've been afraid to go to bed hungry. But, I feel like I've made really big strides in that area. I sleep fine whether I go to bed hungry or not. And if I eat my last food at 9pm and stay up until 1, nothing bad happens. I think I'm ready to switch.

I'm at 209, which is close to Onederland. I only lost 1 pound last week, which seems to me that my loss is slowing on 4&2. So here I go, joining all of you below 1000 calories a day!

June 28: Today blows at work.

A *lot*. Like, an epic lot. Not my fault, but still, horribly stressful.

And, do I want to eat? No. I'm making myself eat because it's time to eat. I had the crab soup at 10:30 because it was filling and yet still liquidy, couldn't handle eating puffs/pretzels/bars or my L&G. Then I had a shake at 1. Still didn't want solid food.

Who am I? Turned a corner here.

June 30: Okay, good to know...

Tonight I changed up my evening ritual, and had crisps instead of dill pickles as my late-night snack. I was hoping that the extra carbs would help with my fuzzy-brained-ness, as suggested by some people on the boards. While the idea may still be spot-on, the timing was epically bad.

It was clear pretty quickly that I was going to eat something off plan. So I had a measured half cup of kim chi. There are worse cheats than 17 calories of cabbage. But I felt very triggered by late-night carbs, and helpless. It wasn't like I was really in control of the act of reaching out for more food. I did keep control over what I grabbed, but not reaching wasn't really an option anymore. Controlled crash...

I don't think I like that feeling. Not one bit.

I am very grateful to be learning more about myself every day on MF. Moral of the story: end the day with fat, protein, and salt, like I usually do (cream cheese and dill pickles), and not with carbs.

4 JULY

July 1: bought more clothes today!

I'm officially out of control. But I was at Costco, and did you know? When you're not a size 22–24 pants and 1x–2x tops, you can buy clothes there! Who knew?

I'm currently 18W pants, XL tops. I have several pairs of 18s and 16s waiting for me to fit into them (but the larger pair of 18s just became "tight but wearable in a pinch" today). So, I bought a pair of 14 jeans. They look so little! And 2 small shirts and a medium dress. I can fit all the shirts/dress onto me now, although they don't look good. But they fit onto my body with varying degrees of comfort.

I am starting to assemble clothing I can wear when my current wardrobe gets too baggy. And things that are smalls should be good for a while, right?

This diet may well be the hardest thing I've ever done. BUT, it sure works. And fitting into those leetle-bitty clothes is so worth it. The Costco samples could not tempt me. I'm worth it.

July 2: those new clothes are going back.

I bought a few new things yesterday at Costco in a burst of excitement. I think I'm taking everything back except for the jeans. Honestly, the clothes aren't that great, and certainly not for 12–18 bucks each. I was just so excited that I could buy normal average clothes in a normal average place.

I have about 6–7 more months OP probably, so I have time to get more clothes. I'm going to build in a regular clearance-rack routine at JC Penney, Nordie's Rack, and Macy's, and see if I can slowly acquire things at rock-bottom prices. This shouldn't be that hard—I can buy anything in a small or medium, which is going to give me a lot of possible clothes. It's a different thing than looking for a decent 1X on a clearance rack—hopeless! Ugly clothes! I'll try to wear the XLs I own until I can start wearing the mediums, and skip buying larges that won't fit at goal.

There is so much learning with this plan! It's not just how to eat, it's also how to build a whole new wardrobe of clothes I'll be happy to wear without breaking the bank.

Oh, and my new belt? The one I bought last weekend? I had to go to the next smaller hole this morning. *squeeee*

July 3: thank you to the smart, smart people on these boards!

I received some excellent advice yesterday from people about not buying goal clothes now, but instead buying them when I'm at or very near goal. They pointed out that my body will change, and styles that look good on me larger won't necessarily look good on me smaller.

So, I'll be taking it all back.

I was going to keep the Gloria Vanderbilt size 14 jeans, but then I pulled out a pair of my old 16s from a few years ago, and guess what? The waistband of the 14s is like an inch *wider* than the 16s I have. I don't need any *bigger* pants than what I already own, I need smaller ones! So, those are going back too, and when my 16s are falling off me I'll go to JC Penney and get a couple pairs of whatever inflated size just barely fits on me. Knowing the way sizes have been going, I'll probably go straight from a loose old 16 to a new 10. *laughing*

Yesterday I went through my entire closet and a large drawer, trying on every single shirt I own. I didn't bother with pants, suits, dresses, because I just wear jeans every day to work and school. But shirts were starting to feel a bit chaotic—I'd try something on and it would be too big, I'd go shopping in the depths and find something too small and finally something just right. All of it was too time-consuming for before work every day. I was tired of wearing the same 6 shirts over and over!

Everything went on and got sorted into "fits now" "fits later" and "already too big" or "ugly." There are a bunch more things in my Goodwill box with the fat pants. My shirts drawer is chock full of things I can wear *right now*, many of them things I haven't worn for a while. And there's one tidy stack in the closet of things I can't wear yet, to fish out the next time things are swimming on me.

Oh! And I tried on *all my bras*. Each and every one of them. One is too big already and in the Goodwill box. A *lot* of others that were too small and uncomfortable are now just fine and peachy. So I think I'm going to transition away from my Decent Exposures all-cotton sports bras (comfortable as heck, but they do not create a good boob profile) and into regular pretty bras. I mean, some of them are gorgeous. I should get some wear out of them before I have to throw them all out. Oooh, and a couple are padded/water bras, and so I'll have ginormous ta-tas. Perhaps even "enter the room before the belly" ta-tas, but that might still be a pipedream.

I switched to 5&1 on Monday. I lost 4 pounds since last Sat. I needed 4&2 in order to learn this program and get through my adjustment phase, but I am glad to see it go if it's going to mean this kind of loss. Wow.

July 4: I made it through yesterday

I feel very pupal. Wrapped up tight in a chrysalis, all squishy and guts and weird rearranging bits of skeleton. Nowhere near ready to step out as who I'm becoming and take on the world. I know that will come, soon enough. But for now, today, I am grateful for my safe little home, in one of the wealthiest nations in the history of time, with clean water to drink, healthy food for my body, the love of my family, safety in my person and possessions, and all the freedom that so many have fought and died to protect.

Bless you all, Bless America, and have a lovely and amazing Fourth.

July 5: good day today

Haven't really heard from my friend, but after the long email I sent yesterday asplainin' my side of things, I feel much more at peace with it. At least I stood up for myself. I've been having a theme in my life lately about being really clear which things I can control and which things I can't, and working on my side of the fence. I guess that's pretty apropos as I'm newly sober about food and that's pretty much the serenity prayer. So, I can control my communication with her, and what I put up with. I can't control her, not one little bit. Letting it go!

Yesterday and today I cleaned. For hours and hours. What with full-time work, law school, being fat and then sick & fat and then fat and then on MF and then finals and then a whirlwind break and then school again—well, let's just say housecleaning hasn't been my highest priority. But I got my things put away. All my floors are vacuumed and scrubbed. Things that don't usually move out of the way to get cleaned under have been cleaned under. The hand wash done. Mold scrubbed off of windowsills. Cat beds laundered. You know, *clean*.

It feels really good. I feel good to have a nice house around me. I feel good that by cleaning off the dining table my spooky-weird kitty will now sleep in her new cat bed. It's on the dining table, you know, because she likes it there. And I feel very good that food has been fine. It hasn't been especially hard this weekend, my first weekend back on 5&1 after 4&2 for 6 weeks or so.

I feel good. It's a good day.

July 6: I missed the window on another shirt

It was too small when I was at my largest. I fished it out last week when I went through my entire closet, trying things on. It fit fine when I first put it on this morning. But after just 2 hours, the "fitted" sash thing around the waist is gapping—like just hanging there, awkwardly. So sad.

Another one for the Goodwill pile when I get home!

And yes—excellent problem to have. I'm okay with it.

July 6: I dream of less "cheatin' talk"

I know everyone's journey is their own, and no one is perfect. I get that. But I am supported by hanging out here with other people who are working hard and suffering along with me, towards the same goal. I experience the opposite of support when I read about people cheating. When they give up on themselves and the plan, it doesn't bolster my will or give me strength.

Do I want people to never share when they've fallen? No. Would I like it a *lot* if they'd focus their posts differently? Yes. I'd love to see cheating posts (when they must appear) that focus on the triggers that led to going off plan, the feelings before/during/after, and the *plan* to get back on track and avoid it in the future. I would like to stop seeing cheating posts that describe in loving detail all the off-plan foods consumed and bemoan the 1.2 pound gain afterwards. Who is that helping, exactly? Is that really what they come here for? What do they think that is doing to support others in the community?

It just feels like going to an AA meeting to talk in living color about last night's margarita party and the hot guy you danced with and how much fun you had. Not the right venue, right?

July 7: I'm the frog in boiling water

Or I was, anyway. You know that thing—if you put a frog into a pot of boiling water, he'll try desperately to get out. If you put a frog in a pot of cold water and gradually increase the temperature, he'll calmly sit there and cook to death.

(Let's leave aside discussions of which circle of hell the person who did this experimenting belongs in...)

Anyway, that was me. Gradually gaining weight. Gradually losing mobility. Gradually having less energy, and less desire to go out, play, and be social. Gradually allowing one bad food/exercise/lifestyle choice to pile on top of another.

I'd think, "I just don't feel like going out tonight." Not letting myself see that I never felt like going out, because I was carting around 100 pounds more than a healthy BMI. 100 pounds! That's like... a lot, dude. A whole frickin' lot. More than a 6th-grader.

I did the same thing with a friendship—just let myself coast down into her depression zone with her. Our "adventures" ceased, and became just sitting in the hot tub, and then mostly phone calls. All the fun had left the relationship, and I didn't notice because it was so gradual.

Well, she's decided to take a break from talking to me, and I'm discovering how much lighter I feel for not having to help carry that weight of sadness every day. I have a family member with some severe depression/medication issues who I've elected to step away from until they get some of that turned around. When my friend stopped calling, I had the thought—well, now I've got room to pick up that family member now.

Hell no! Just because I'm not weighed down to the maximum amount of misery I can stand doesn't mean I should look around for more misery to fill my dance card with. Where the hell did that thought come from? I screamed my defiance the whole way home. I am so grateful for cars and freeways for unobserved crazy-person emotional processing.

I choose something different. I choose not to go back in the pot. I choose to reach out to friends who nurture me, who bring me joy and adventure and *fun*. I choose to invest in myself now.

I am turning this around. Now. Today, and tomorrow, and one white packet at a time. I'm cleaning house and resisting the urge to go ask the neighbors if I can move their trash into my living room.

July 8: Eeek! I'm all askeered!

deep breath Okay, today will be a momentous occasion. I should set the stage: it's *hawt* in Seattle right now. High of 90 today, which should be right about as I'm heading to class. I'm already wearing a tank top, which is by itself a little nerve-wracking. *But*, I plan to make it ever so much worse and...

Wear. Cute. Shoes.

ZOMG! *faint*

I don't know if I've ever worn cute shoes to school before. They're just sandals, but they have a high heel and a zipper—they're the ones I blogged about a month ago if you recall. I'm actually nervous. I'm nervous to do it. Sexy shoes say something different about you. They're not over the line or anything—I have plenty of classmates who wear similar shoes. But it's new for me.

So, wish me luck. And courage. And maybe keep your fingers crossed that today could be the day that someone finally says something.

giggle

July 8: Update on the shoes...

Well, I wore them. It felt mostly good, and a little exposed. However, I need not have worried about exposed, as still... not a peep.

I am going to start stabbing classmates in the eye with a highlighter screaming "Maybe if you just have one eye you'll use it more wisely!" Seriously. Don't they realize it's time for them to do a little work—namely *noticing me*???!?!!?! What could be more important?

sigh

It's about 3 blocks of walking each way, although there's a lot of sky bridge and corridor nonsense involved. It was enough that I found out where the shoe rubs on my left foot—a patch of skin between the size of a chicken-noodle-soup "chicken" chunk and the size of a beef stew "pea" is now missing. Ah well, it was good to break the ice on the new shoes, the concept of hottie heels, and a tank top with a damn fine bra. Which BTW did not leave my rib cage with a painful bruise. It actually fit.

In other news, I attempted my first truly improvisational move with the MF food, and while I would not inflict it on anyone else, it did actually still hit the spot. I wanted something solid/savory, had had pretzels 2.5 hours ago, and was out of all cream soups. I tossed a beef stew in the blender to dustify it, and then more or less used Kurz's bagel recipe, except that I made muffins. Turns out it made some dry bland little muffins, but hey... what do I care? I have to drink tons of water anyway, and I'll eat cardboard if you tell me it's OP.

Hope everyone is having a lovely amazing OP night!

July 9: I am eating...

... the other half of my batch of dry flavorless lumpy little beef-stew biscuit turds this morning for snack. No pride whatsoever.
That is all.

July 10: A friend just cancelled our plans for today...

... and I'm just glad that I don't have to rearrange my food schedule for today.
Life's little gifts! Downside: being at home alone instead of being social. Upside: more time to study, and I don't have to eat L&G before I want it so I have more MF meals in my purse as we gad about. Oh, and other upside: more time on the boards with ya'all that I don't have to feel is taking away from studying.
I'll take it.

July 12: today blows

My heart is breaking a little. 2 weeks since my best friend spoke to me. She falls into these pits of depression, and not gracefully, and suddenly the person I talk to twice a day is just gone gone gone...
I am hungry, but not wanting to eat off plan. This, at least, is a blessing.
I'd like this to hurt less so I can concentrate at work. I really suck today.

July 13: State of the Union

I feel like I have a lot swirling around inside me, and I just want to list it all out somewhere.
Crappy things:

- work has some serious leadership issues, and I'm burnt out and struggling

- still haven't talked to my friend, and that's slightly worrisome (not hugely worrisome since I got a voicemail, so that's a big improvement)
- I'm deeply, *deeply* bored with the MF food right now. I'm sure I'm learning something important about food-as-fuel, but ugh. It's like I don't even care what packet I grab. I'm going to be hungry and unsatisfied no matter what I eat, so who cares?
- this feels like an eternal process. Like eternal. And there's a part of me that's very frightened of long-term maintenance, like all the fun will have been sucked out of the universe forever.
- I'm still fat! All this hard work, and still fat! Also, a weird little bulgy place between my boobs where I'm losing fat unevenly. Also other unpleasant places on my body as the stomach starts to sag a little. Ick.
- Scale says 203...203...203... Onederland *mocks me*.
- Still in the two pairs of 18Ws, which are starting to feel like the Pants of Purgatory. *booming voice* "You Shall Wear These Saggy-Butt Pants Until You *Die In Them Mwahahahahaha!*"

Good things:

- I am healthy and reasonably happy day-to-day
- my house is all fantastically awesomely clean because I have more MFing energy
- summer term is over in 2 weeks and then I get 3.5 weeks of blissful break
- I lost 33 pounds in 2.5 months
- I get to go to a regional Burning Man festival with 500 people frolicking in the woods in 2 weeks, for 3 days (during study days for my exam, so that's going to be hilarious.)
- I just got a Board position on the Law Review because someone resigned. It's the job I wanted, and I kept campaigning for it even after I wasn't selected a couple months ago, because I just *knew* it was my job. It's source checking for LR articles, and I get to build giant forts out of library books and catch authors' sloppy little plagiarisms and

I love it. It also gives me 3 credits for LR for this year instead of 1, which is pretty much a whole other exam I never have to take.
- I am in possession of the first couple disks of ER Season 13—yay Netflix!
- I have all ya'all for help and support
- I am reaching out to lots of other people and gradually making plans with them—leaving the best-friend-bunker-of-sadness
- despite boredom and the process seeming eternal, I don't actually want to go off plan at all. It's not really even a consideration.
- I believe, yup, pretty sure, that I received some male attention yesterday. Guy was flirting his butt off at the eyeglasses store. Not someone I was into, but it was nice that it happened.

Enuf for now…

July 14: I don't recognize my hands…

From yesterday to today, I don't recognize my hands. My fingers got skinnier, and apparently I just noticed. My wrist bones, too. Weird.

Holding steady at 202, but I'm in the larger pair of size 18s. Just in time, too, as one of the 2 pairs of Purgatory Pants just developed a rip by a pocket. So, I still have only 2 pairs of wearable pants, but one actually fits me well.

I exercised my new superpower last night—indifference to food. I met a friend for a drink after class. Normally I would want something that would stay with me as my last meal—a brownie, a bagel, or soup. Bars are too sweet and don't make me feel full. But, I just told myself that fundamentally I was going to be hungry and unsatisfied no matter what I ate, so it didn't matter. I had mint tea and a PB bar while she had a glass of wine and dessert. And I was fine. I stayed on my food schedule and enjoyed being social.

Went home and had my dill pickles and went to bed hungry. Again. Because I have that superpower now too.

Feeling pretty darned good.

July 14: math

11 weeks down. 33 pounds. 3 pounds, on average, week after week after week for almost 3 months.

I rawk. MF rawks. I rawk MF.

In even better news, my big order arrived today and I have a raspberry brownie in the freezer waiting for me to take it to school with me. And I get to make bagels for dinner. *Yum!*

July 18: Yay for festival on Thursday!

Lots going on here in my life. My friend is talking to me again, and all seems well. We've hung out twice, for about an hour, just easing back into things again. It's a goodness.

I am starting to like things nice and tight around my waist. I used to find any sort of pressure annoying and uncomfortable. Now I keep cinching my belt tighter, because it feels good and secure. Of course, that the belt fastens on the 5th hole now, when 3 weeks ago I was on the first—that's not just me enjoying things tighter. That's my fat leaving my body and things compacting themselves into place like good body parts. Yay, body!

I was a bridesmaid yesterday—posted a pic of me in that silly dress on my page. The poor dress never had a chance—I lost 35 pounds between ordering it and the wedding. I had dropped enough weight in the last 2 weeks that the alterations were totally off, too. Didn't get it anywhere near fitting right. We had to put a row of safety pins up one side to keep it from horribly gapping.

By the time I'd been in it for 6 hours I thought it was hilarious and wore it to another party after the reception. A BBQ/housewarming. In a bridesmaid's dress. It was hilarious and awesome. I cut out my head for my new avatar pic, because I really have a whole lot fewer chins. Like a lot. Kinda cool.

I did really good around all the food. Rehearsal dinner, wedding dinner, BBQ food. I just ignored all of it like it didn't exist. Except for the wedding dinner which was pizza and salads. I had a little internal struggle about the beet salad—*beets!* I love them so much! Oh, and it was family style, so I had to pass every single dish as it went around the table. There was a pizza with a stray piece of bacon. You know, a neglected little orphan that had fallen off a piece someone else took, and was just sitting all alone. I was actually paralyzed for a minute holding that plate staring at that piece of bacon. But, eventually I managed to hand the plate to the bride and get back to my PB crunch bar. Which I had unwrapped and placed on my plate, and ate as slowly as possible.

Yesterday I saw 6 people I'd been to Mexico with in Feb. *Not one word.* I sweartagod it's a conspiracy. There's someone walking around ahead of me telling everyone "Don't say anything about the weight Freya lost. You know, it's because of that horrible vaginal rash she has—she's been squirming around so much it's made her lose a bunch of weight and she's horribly self-conscious about it. So not a word, okay?" Because otherwise, it makes no sense. 35 pounds, people!

I just spent like 4 hours in the kitchen prepping food for the week and for camping. I made a dozen bagel/muffins. 8 brownies in different flavors: mint, orange, cheesecake, coffee, coconut. I made salads for the next few days, and turkey with egg beaters. For camping, I have chicken I'll put into 3 ounce ziplocs. And I made a really simple gazpacho (fresh tomatoes, cucs, and bell peppers, with salt, blended in Cuisinart) which is amazingly good and I hope still edible after freezing: 1.5 cups in each container. It'll thaw gradually and make a lovely cold slushy green. Oh, and 5 water bottles of pink lemonade Crystal Light are in the freezer as well.

Feeling pretty good. A lot of social fun, really good physical energy, food's ready for camping... I'm tired and a little headachy from yesterday being such a big day. My Evidence exam is in 8 days and we have to do a presentation tomorrow in class, and so far I'm *screwed* for both. But hey—at least I look good. And there are 8 more days!

Hope everyone is having an amazing OP day!

July 22: off I go... camping for 3 days...

Well, I finish up with work in a couple hours. Then I go to class. Then back to work to print out my final class notes and leave my computer locked up safe, and not with me in the woods. Then I head an hour+ north to the camp site, and sleep in my car! I bought a Buick Rendezvous and it's got plenty of room for my double-bed futon in the back, so I just toss my stuff into the front seats and curl up snuggly. Of course, this will be after a couple/few hours of wandering around saying hello to people and hanging out.

I'll be there until Sunday afternoon. Since today started early (to finish packing) and will go late, I'm modifying my food today, Friday, and Saturday. I'm having 2 cheese sticks in addition to my regular food. I'll split my lean and have 3 oz of chicken + a cheese stick at lunch time, and the same at dinner time. Just a little extra protein to support me through all the walking around.

Otherwise, it's the regular 5&1 in the woods! Bagels, brownies, pretzels, bars... Chicken & gazpacho. Cream cheese and dill pickles. Hooray!

Wish me luck with studying! My final is on Monday so I'm supposed to spend part of my time working my brain in a camp chair while in the woods. Ha! (No really, that's what I'll be doing. Really.)

Oh, and I'm stuck in Twoderville until at least Monday. No scale in the woods, and this morning it mocked me with *200 200 200* some more. Little bastid.

July 25: 100% OP while camping and surrounded by bacon!

3 days in the woods camping with 500 or so of my closest friends. My "camp" had maybe 15–20 people in it—I never got entirely clear on who was camping with us and who was just around a lot—it never seemed to matter. Anyway, many of them were cooking much of the time. It's pretty safe to say that I could smell bacon cooking for about 6 hours of Saturday, from my camp or others nearby.

So many delights were offered to me, and I passed them all up. Not one BLT [Bites Licks, and Tastes] of any kind. Hooray!

I stuck to my plan of 5&1 + 2 cheese sticks + 1T cream cheese extra (this was a late addition after I miscalculated my healthy fat allotment the first night and decided it was a good idea anyway.) So I ran around 1050 calories/day. There was a *lot* of up hill and over dale, and dancing both Thurs and Fri nights. Today I'm back to regular 5&1, no extras, because there was only a little morning dancing and packing up to leave, but not any significant exertions. I lived entirely on brownies and muffins—didn't eat a single one of the bars or pretzels I brought.

Tomorrow morning we see if pesky old Onederland has made an appearance, or if the groundhog is going back in its burrow for 6 more weeks of fattier-ness.

I'm sunburnt and bug bitten, but I'm happy with the amount of studying I did from a camp chair and feel well-rested. In 26 hours my exam starts and in 30 it's over and I get 3.5 weeks off!

PS in case you're keeping track—Still. Not. One. Single. Word. It's a conspiracy of silence!

July 27: Why 100% OP is the most peaceful food choice I've ever made...

Yes, it's hard. Absurdly hard sometimes, like for the entire first 6 weeks. *laughing* But now I'm 3 months in, and things have shifted. For the most part, I'm floating through my days, almost effortlessly OP. I can ignore a plate of bacon passed to me (well, I smell it lovingly, but my fingers don't want to reach), pass by a buffet table without a 2nd thought, and eat a bar while others eat pizza.

For me, that is entirely the result of staying 100% OP. Every day, I eat my MF foods and my similar, simple L&Gs. My food is not exciting, it's fuel. It tastes amazing to me because my taste buds are all cleaned out. But most importantly, I can largely silence the greedy food monster by not following its "suggestions." When the voices of rationalization say I should have a little of that because I'm tired or it's been a long day or I walked around a lot at the mall, I have ignored them for 3 months straight. And at some point, they started to give up and get weak... wispy faint rationalizing voices... while the voice of "I just stay OP all the time because that's what I do" has grown rowdy-strong and powerful.

Yesterday was a challenging day. I had to take a 3.5 hour law school exam from 6:30–10PM. That's full-tilt high-functioning balls-to-the-wall reading, writing, and ZOMG pretty late at night. I ate my last MF meal at 8 during the exam. After, I went for drinks with a couple classmates to chill out a bit. They had beer and fries. I had a mint tea. I didn't consider eating any fries—they are not for me. I got home around 12:30 and had 2 dill pickles and 1T of cream cheese, my remaining OP food for the day. It was 3:30am before the afternoon's green tea and the general excitement of exam day wore off enough for me to sleep.

Not once in there did I seriously consider having something "extra" to get me through. I knew my hunger was not an emergency, that at 8:30 the next morning I'd have a shake, and that I was out of food for the day. I enjoyed the tummy rumbling and didn't really think about it much.

That's the liberation of not deviating from the plan. It sets me free. It gives me back control. It allows me to learn a new place inside me, and that new place will be what allows me to find and follow a workable food plan long-term.

July 29: "Pick what OP means for you and stick to it 100%"

When I say that, do I mean have a KFC double-down every Sunday or add fruit to your yogurt? No, that's not what I mean. What I mean is that most of us have an emotional relationship with food that is not working for us (obviously excepting people who ate the same thing for 40 years and then a medication or health issue caused them to gain weight). With all of our emotional and mental attachments to food, we have a whole lot of voices in our heads.

There's the voice of the addict. It wants *more more more*. It thinks it needs food for comfort, or to quiet anger, or to alleviate boredom. It imagines that going to bed a little hungry could *kill me by morning* OMG!

There's the voice of the practical, "I have to live my life" side of ourselves. That part acknowledges that our job requires eating out frequently, or that doing without Laughing Cow or peanut butter would be the one step too far that would make us give up on the plan entirely.

There's the voice of our new, emerging wisdom that knows which choices are healthy ones. The voice that can listen to the other inputs and weed out the garbage from the healthy. The small, quiet, neglected, almost completely powerless voice when we start, that grows in strength each and every day we stay 100% OP.

So how do we deal with all these voices? We need to strengthen the wisdom, honor the practical, and shut down the addict. This is a different process for everyone. MF gives a basic structure, but the exact combination of things that will accomplish that for me is not the same combination that will do it for someone else.

My addict thinks that 4 oz of LF cheddar melted over roasted peppers sounds like a perfectly awesome L&G. My addict looks at the list of condiments and says "So I can have 3T of LF cream cheese and 2T of full-fat cream cheese each and every day if I want? Or put 3T of parmesan in a pan and fry it up to get crispy?" Yes, the plan allows that. No, I will not be eating that way. Someone else may manage their addict voice by avoiding PB flavored things, or not eating all brownies all day, or staying away from snack-food-ish things. We all have to find our own path to not indulge the addict—because believe me, we can indulge it even within the confines of the plan!

What about honoring the practical? For each of us, there are things that, while not coming from the addict, are nonetheless not negotiable. I will not give up or even restrict my salt intake. I won't count condiments. Someone else won't give up eating in restaurants (and will not bring a scale and measuring cup either), or an extra stick of string cheese when really hungry, or half and half in morning coffee regardless of whether they have a healthy fat for it that day. Those sort of choices are based on an honest recognition that practicalities exist, and we have to make our peace with the plan. A functional, livable peace.

Then we use the voice of wisdom to craft our own plan. For me, well, those condiments... Do I let myself go hog-wild because I don't obsessively count them? No. I have one simple rule, and a closed universe of options. My rule is that I shed them whenever possible. If I've been putting LorAnne oils in my shakes for a while, I try them without. Oh look, I don't care if there's another flavor in my dark chocolate shake anymore! So I do without. Same thing with salad dressing—one day I tried it without and found I didn't miss it, and now I don't eat it anymore. My closed universe? I eat only the following condiments and no others: PAM, dried spices, salt, hot sauce, bouillon, extracts, baking powder. As a further restriction to make up for a day when I might have 2tsp of bouillon and 1 baking powder and some garlic powder—I restrict my optional snack. I only eat dill pickles, never something with more fat or carbs.

My plan is slightly different from your plan. It always will be. Am I jealous that someone else can eat all that melted cheese? Sure. But then again, there's probably someone jealous of me that I could eat 5 brownies in a day and be just fine. We all have to find our own road, with wisdom managing practicality and shutting down the addict.

July 30: No more pancakes for my inner addict. Also pants.

Well, I'm onto that little trollop. I had acknowledged that the pancakes just make me really, no I mean *really* want butter. But this week I caught myself deciding the other side of the pancake really needed its own spray of butter-flavored PAM. And then there was just an unholy amount of pleasure at the one little bit of edge that had enough PAM to be crispy.

Forget it. I am clearly not up to the challenges of pancakes. *grin* Took them back out of my next order. I'll finish this one box, but no more...

In pants news, wow is it dismal in my closet. I have fit into the smallest pair of 18s comfortably enough to wear them. The 18Ws fit 5 belt loops ago, and they're held up by the magic of a strip of leather. But now they've started to shred. One of the 18Ws has developed a couple rips, one of which is located in the rear of my rear, and so is totally unwearable. The smallest pair, the ones that fit the best, I discovered while wearing them yesterday is close to shredded where the thighs rub together, with enough actual holes to be unwearable. I guess I didn't evaluate the vitality of my smaller pants before I tucked them away in the closet on my way up.

Soooo... I bought a pair of 12s and 14s in the Gloria Vanderbilt stretch line at Costco yesterday. I wanted to try on the 14s and see how close I am before buying 16s. Not close enough, but 16s should do it. I can't be wearing only 2 pairs of sad, pathetic, droopy-butted pants day after day after day, it's making me crazy! I'll be back there today, to get some 16s, try them on in the bathroom, and if they're the winners I think they will be, buy a second pair *right that minute*.

A girl's gotta live. And I just can't take looking at my elephant-dropped-load tookus in the mirror all the time!

July 30: I started telling them NO!

Today was the first... I wrote back to a Nordstrom's email about a sale on plus size clothes, and told them I am no longer plus-sized and to please update my demographics in their email system.

Hooray!

Next up, some phone calls to Jessica London and such. I'd say "later" but I mean "never"!

July 31: State of the Union

40 pounds down, in 3 months. 27.5 inches between the various things we log on this site, including 8 from my waist alone.

From size 24Ws to size 16s. Same brand of jeans, too—those were GV stretch 24s, and they're GV stretch 16s. So no size inflation there—that's for reals 4 full sizes down.

New pics of the 16s on my page. A little muffin-toppy still, but I'll wear them with looser shirts for the next, what, week? Two? Until that goes away. I've attached one of them here, too.

I love this diet. With deep gratitude to MF and this wonderful community and to that which makes all things possible...

5 AUGUST

August 2: This is freaking me out now

This morning as I looked at the scale, I thought "Oh no, not another one..." I was overwhelmed that it had gone down another pound. That's 6 into Onederland, and I just arrived here 6 days ago.

But it's also the cumulative thing. 41 pounds, into size 16s... It's the changes in my body—everywhere I look something new. When I flex my calf there's a ridge of bone and a dimple in the muscle. There's a lumpy place in my belly fat where a pocket isn't shrinking as fast as what's around it. There are bones and lines of muscle emerging everywhere. I can sit with my legs crossed.

It's also an emotional thing. A fear thing. Size 16s are what I was wearing when I met the last boyfriend. The Epic Love boyfriend. The Sociopathic Con Artist Married boyfriend (I didn't know any of that until 3 years after we broke up... but it still hurt my soul deeply...) Now I'm at a weight where men register my presence everywhere I go. I'm not saying they come up and ask me out, but they *see* me, in a way they didn't 3 months ago.

3 months. It's sooooo fast. I'm not getting off the train, but wow. I am feeling the Mach forces today.

August 4: Conscious Denial = My Friend

Well, it's day 3 of the Denial Plan. I am officially in my head *not losing any more weight*. I weigh 197 and that's IT. I'm a size 18, too.

(Nevermind what the scale may have said in the past or could say now—or whether I happen to be wearing size 16 pants or not—the scale is in the closet and that's that.)

I'm sticking with denial until I don't feel so overwhelmed by the crazy changes. I am really freaked out, for 3 days now, which is a long time for one mood for me! About 50 times a day I reassure myself, "It's okay. I'm still fat. Nice and fat. Big belly. Squish it, it's huge." Then I look down and stick it out, or pooch it out and look at myself sideways if there's a mirror handy. Yup, fat. Phew!

Trying to let my brain catch up to my body. Staying 100% OP, so yeah, the body is probably continuing to do its thing while I pretend it's not. But you can't make me notice. And "OP" is just what I eat, NOT a "diet." Because that would imply losing weight, which I am *not doing lalalalalala!*

Tomorrow, baggy sweats (thanks, Chris!).

So fat! Staying fat! It's safe here and I'm not leaving!

August 27: Stay out of the Plus Size Section, girl!

You don't belong here!

Well, it sunk in emotionally this morning, what I found out a couple weeks ago. I went shopping for professional blouses. Out of habit, or thinking that it was where I belonged, I went to the Women's sections. Everything was way too big. I finally found one blouse in a 0X that I purchased.

Then I went to the regular section, "just in case," to see if they might have something... you know... cut extra-large or something. Well, the XLs there fit perfectly. I got home and tried on that 0X again and it gapped at the armpits and had to be returned.

It's official. I am no longer welcome in the fat lady section. They have nothing for me there. At 186 I'm wearing 16 jeans, 18 dress suit, and XL blouses. 0X is too big.

This feels like a loss of an old friend. An old friend with whom I had an unhealthy relationship. *wink* Relief, gladness to be free, and some sadness to leave the familiar behind.

Luckily I have a new friend greeting me with open arms. Hooray!

August 28: Smells...

I've been totally huffing molecular carb clouds lately. My coworker heated up rice in the nuker and I would take deep breaths all the way down the hall, filled with pleasure at the aromas of carbs. As he microwaved yesterday's pasta, he poked his head in my office and asked if I was going to need to smell his lunch today. *laughing* Oops. Busted.

Last night I was out with a couple friends for massages. We were done at 10pm, and then stopped at a minimart, and then the two of them wanted to get diner food. They were going to have me drop them off. I was out of food for the day (except for my pickles "nightcap"), and had last eaten at 8 so I was working towards physically hungry again. And I realized that partly I wanted their company, and partly I really *really* wanted to huff some greasy diner food.

Thank goodness they're indulgent kind people. They may have laughed at me, but they raised no objections as I smelled pancakes, sausages, bacon, ham, hash browns, toast, whipped cream, and hot cocoa. Everything smelled so good!

I sipped my herbal tea. And then I checked in with myself. I wasn't suffering. I didn't have any urges or cravings to put any of their food in my mouth. I wasn't having to sit on my hands or in any way fight down demons. I was truly enjoying the smells of the food and that was actually all I wanted.

Miracles. I love MF.

August 30: No reserves

I've been coming to the conclusion that MF doesn't leave me much in the way of reserves. This makes sense, right? It puts us in the gray area between "eating enough calories to sustain life" and "total metabolic shutdown." This is not the body's preferred zone. It likes "enough calories" better.

Sometimes I have those bursts of energy, I do. And I always have more energy than I did when I was carting 49 more pounds around—that's a *lot*. But, I don't handle challenges as well as I would like to.

PMS? Devastating. Painful, exhausting, uncomfortable, unpleasant.

Stress? Exhausting. I need more time than I usually would to cope with the challenges in my life.

My kitchen being covered in plastic for a week when it should have been 2 days? It's thrown off everything else in my life, as the mess has spilled out into every other room of the house.

When things are going well, I have a lot more "in the zone" feelings than I did when so much fatter. When things are not going well, I just feel flattened.

Anyone else? How do you experience this? Feel you have less in your reserve tanks?

6 SEPTEMBER

September 5: Well that was cool

I was invited to a wedding tonight. I knew it was a sit-down catered thing, because the reply card asked me to choose from beef, fish, chicken, and vegetarian entrée. I knew I would want to eat enough to be polite, and I knew I'd have *zero* control over what showed up on my plate.

In that, I was correct. It was the big catered thing where everyone gets the same thing. I had bars in my purse, but I really didn't want to ignore my entire plate of food and scurry off to eat a bar in the bathroom.
But it worked out really well!
I eat my L&G at 1:00 and I didn't want to show up there super hungry, in case it was like a plate of pasta with an ounce of beef or some other disaster. So I ate my regular L&G at 1:00 and planned to have a 4&2 day, assuming I could eat there.
The appetizers were crab salad on lettuce leaves, olives, radishes, and cheese crackers. I ignored all of it. I knew the food would have enough fats that I would not need any olives. The salad was romaine, hearts of palm, avocado, and grapefruit with a vinaigrette. I pushed the avocado and grapefruit off to the side with my poor abandoned roll, and tried not to cry over the avocado. That was the only hard moment. That avocado *really* wanted to ride on up to my mouth on my fork.

The entrée was a big piece of beef with a sauce on/under it, on a bed of potatoes and chanterelles, with carrots on the side. I excavated the beef, pushing everything under and on it off to the side as casually as I could, and enjoyed the heck out of what was probably 6 ounces of steak. And I picked out the like 5 1/2 inch wide chanterelles.

I logged it as 6 ounces of steak, 1.5 cups of romaine, and 2.5 tsp of canola oil (as I have no way to tell exactly how much fat was in the salad dressing or left on the steak after scraping). I'm skipping the 2 healthy fats I am "owed" from lunch. And with how I have it logged, it comes out to 1133 calories, which is def. within the 1000–1200 guidelines for 4&2.

I am counting this as a total win. I didn't eat any off-plan foods. I did *chill out* and let the food that was served be okay. I ate out for the 2nd time in over 4 months since I started MF, and the world did not end.

Oh, and I had a good time at the wedding.

September 8: yup—anger is one of my triggers

Well, so far I had identified loneliness/emptiness as the major feeling that makes me want to eat. I thought anger was not high up on that list, as generally when I'm angry I just go pace around the block on the phone with my BFF.

But, I think maybe that's for the easy kind of anger—the quick shallow PO'd kind. Right now I'm having some deep abiding frustrated anger about a long-standing situation that is taking some time and care to extricate myself from. It's been extra up for me the last couple days. Guess what? They've been "hungry days" where I've eaten my meals earlier than scheduled.

Well, today I spent 2.5 hours on the extrication project, and wow. Now I'm not too hungry anymore. Phew.

Learning all the time... So glad I have my obsessive dedication to the plan. If I didn't have that, I would have eaten a massive plate of something to calm myself down, and I wouldn't have learned what I learned today.

Once again, thanks MF!

September 13: I think I'm over the hump

I've lost 55 pounds, with 30-ish left to go. Which you would think meant more than halfway there, right? But weight loss slows when you have less to lose.

I lost 3 pounds a week for the first 12 weeks. Then I lost 2.375/week for the next 8 weeks. I've been on MF for 20 weeks now. If I can keep losing 2/week, I'll be at goal in 15 weeks. If it's 2/week for 11 weeks and 8 weeks at 1/week, I'll be at goal in 19 weeks. Which seems pretty darned attainable even as a pessimistic estimate.

So, I'm more than halfway there in terms of time. If I just did 20 weeks without death ensuing, surely I can do 15–19 more, right? As long as Costco keeps stocking egg beaters I should be okay.

Hope everyone is having a lovely day!

September 16: Feeling emotional today

Stirred up... Let's see... I've been a little sick for a week, just enough to take the edge off everything and make it all less fun. I'm down to 180, which feels like a significant number.

180 is the number in my head associated with how I ballooned up in high school. I weighed around 180 when the mean boys sat in the back of 6th period and mooed at me. Mooed. So I'm now *down* to the "active cruelty" point for high school boys.

At the same time, 180 represents this amazing loss of 55 pounds, and I look pretty fantastic. I'm getting flirted with and *seen* in a way I wasn't a few short months ago. I'm fitting into almost every cute thing in my closet. So it's weird to have these opposite impressions of this number.

15 years ago I weighed 130–135 in an abusive relationship. When I left, I gained 60 pounds in a year or two. I needed some defenses! So at 180, I'm also back inside the "danger zone" psychologically. And getting closer and closer to the weight where bad things happen.

Obviously weighing less doesn't mean bad things will happen now—I know that. But the body has its own memory and its own fears, and these feelings are stirred up by the changes in my body. I have a feeling that's why I'm so hungry and bloated this week. I touched 180 on Sunday morning, and I've been between 181.5 and 182.5 every morning since. And my pants are tighter than they were last week—pure bloat as I've been OP and am not constipated. It's not PMS, either... I think it's just fear.

That's cool. I was pretty stressed by it when I weighed 200 for 10 days straight. But now I'm a little more used to the body reacting to a number and putting the brakes on while it decides it's okay to move forward again. I'll stay OP, and eventually we'll all be moving forward together.

Hope everyone is having a lovely OP day...

September 21: Holy NSVs, Batman!

Yesterday was a really good day. Over the weekend I found this great skirt at Ross for $8.00. Knee-length, lining out of dark gold shiny fabric, black floral lace over it. Pretty. So I wore stockings, 3" heels with some patent leather shiny, a form-fitting black silk knit tank, and a little jacket with a fake fur collar.

I was *smokin'* compared to the jeans and big shirts, tennis-shoe-wearing, slouchy fat woman who was prowling the halls of campus a few short months ago.

First of all, I wore those heels *all day long* and didn't even mind. In fact, I'm wearing them again today with jeans. My knees don't hurt at all. This is heaven. Just heaven. Cute shoes!

Then, there were classmates telling me how pretty I looked. I was talking to 3 people, 2 of which I hadn't seen in a while. They asked why I was so dressed up. I said, "I'm just celebrating being less fat." Which prompted lots of laughter and then the ice was broken. "How are you doing it?" "I didn't recognize you!" etc.

I get to my next class, and after class someone tells me "we were talking about you during class. About how skinny you are."

It was a good day. I felt like Jackie Kennedy with my stockings and little fur collar.

September 22: Dancing

I went two-stepping tonight. I haven't been partner dancing in I don't know how many years. I was partnered up with a good strong lead for the lesson, and then he and I danced a couple two-steps.

It was wonderful. I'm rusty, for sure. But there were moments when I felt sassy and light on my feet and trusting his lead... There were times when I closed my eyes while two-stepping. That's one of my favorite things, ever, anywhere.

After an hour and a half I felt overwhelmed and had to run away home. I have all this sadness too, about the years I wasted not being able to dance. About having decided that egg rolls were more important than dancing. They're not, you know. They're just really not.

I thank God for the opportunity to remember who I am.

September 24: I've been hungry for 5 months

It's kind of impressive, really. There has not been a single day in 5 months when I haven't been hungry a good portion of it. I have gone to bed hungry every night for 150 nights. I am still hungry after almost all of my meals, and physically hungry for the hour before each meal. Even when an L&G is physically filling, it's extremely rare for me not to have the "okay, sure, but can I get an appetizer with this, or seconds, or could something in it be fried?" feeling.

5 months of hunger. There is a fleeting little not-very-powerful voice that is bugging me with "isn't this enough already? You can go dancing, your new Calvin Klein dress is a 14, people tell you you look amazing, your knees don't hurt, why not stop?" I'm choosing to ignore it and stay OP until *I'm* good and done.

Because if I can be hungry for 5 months, I can be hungry for 8–9 months. And then there's transition and maintenance. Which bring beets, yogurt, and Dave's Killer Bread. Also about 1500–1750 calories, if my activity level is what I expect it to be. And after 900, 1700 sounds like a *lot*.

So I'm hanging in here. But I want it noted for the record, I'm hungry. Sometimes mentally hungry, sometimes emotionally hungry, a whole lot of the time physically hungry. It's a pretty strange existence after what I did previously. Pretty darned strange...

September 26: Admitting I'm just one Super Woman, not two...

I would say "admitting I'm not Super Woman," but really, I have a full-time job and I'm 4th in my class in law school, which I attend in the evenings, and I've just lost 58 pounds while in school. I think it's okay if I claim one "Super Woman" by my name.

But, I don't have to try for two. I have a big change I want to make. A change that will result in a whole lot of mental challenge and long hours. A change that will require sustained energy levels and mental acuity.

Mental acuity. Therein is my problem. I'm not *dumb* on 5&1. But I'm also not as sharp as I am when I'm eating more than 85g carbs/900 calories. Even after 5 months, I feel, all day long, every day, that my brain is in a little bit of a fog. Sustained focus is pretty much impossible. Even after eating a big L&G.

It makes sense to me. I mean, on 900 calories a day, the body is like, "Brain, if you're going to go being such an incompetent dumbass as to put us on starvation rations like this, well, we'll give you enough juice to kill a bison but if you think you're going to discover algebra right now you can just forget it. Go kill that bison. *Stat*." I just think my brain's on a budget.

I also have the information that a lot of other people have reported this phenomenon when we discuss it on the boards. So I'm not doing anything wrong, I'm just experiencing one of the side-effects of sustained mild ketosis. And it's worth it to me to put up with this to get to goal.

So I decided to wait. The major huge demanding life change can wait until I can eat 1500 or 1750 calories a day. It can wait until I remove the 5&1 from my life, thereby clearing space for this new thing to still fall inside the "One Super Woman" metric, not push me over to two. This is hard on me, on my "I can do it! I'm still trying to earn my father's love!" self. But I'm learning, slowly, to admit my limitations and plan accordingly.

Through the end of the year: full-time work, law school, 5&1, whatever personal/emotional work goes along with my food issues, two-stepping, shopping for cute clothes and enjoying high heels.

Sometime in the spring: full-time work, law school, T&M, new challenge.

I think it'll be okay.

September 28: Lowering goal weight

Screw it! I've been thinking "I'll leave it at 150 until I get to 150, and then I'll lower it." But I've been haunted by this wonderful thing someone said on the boards a couple weeks ago—"Just because I got up to [235] doesn't mean I have to settle for 150."

And there you have it. I want to be a small person, without this big gut hanging out in front. I'm only 5'2". The MF site recommends 118 for me as a mid-range of healthy goal weight. So screw it. I feel better about aiming for 140. We'll see what it looks like when I get there, or closer, and of course I reserve the right to call "goal" at 152 or 137 or whatever. But I was tired of looking at 150 on my ticker and feeling like a coward.

So there you have it. New goal on ticker. Hear me roar.

September 28: Frickin' butt bones

I just walked to the store because I couldn't stand my (padded) desk chair one minute longer. I have these tender little baby butt bones that just hurt when I sit on them!

I found I was curling over to shift my weight so I wasn't on those bones. Well, my posture should not be subject to such indignities. I now have an extra fluffy pillow to put under my delicate ass.

Oh. My. God.

7 OCTOBER

October 4: Fat and glum about it

Body image issues, anyone? Right now I feel 100 times more unattractive than I did when I started MF. At least before I started I was fat and fine with it, hanging with my fat-positive friends, and being social at events that revolved around food.

Now I've dropped 60 pounds, I'm still 11 pounds away from not being OBESE anymore, and I'm hating my body. I have this spider belly that just won't quit. I've been in the same size 16 jeans for 21 pounds, and the camel toe in the 14s is not relenting any time soon. Shifting my focus from "loving myself as I am" to "working so hard to lose weight" has landed me in a really unpleasant mood about my body right now.

I've lost that sexy feeling. I'm sure it'll come back. I just miss it right now. Bleh.

I've been thinking a lot about Corbie's post about goal weight. I loved what she said, all of it. The thing about how after you've been maintaining for a while the glow of comparing yourself to the obese person you were will have worn off, and you'll regret it if you don't get to a goal weight that's healthy for you... Not settling. It's a wonderful insight, and I'm grateful she said it. But emotionally, it seems to have (at least temporarily) stripped away the "ZOMG I'm so skinny!" goggles I was wearing, and left me with "in reality-land, not in comparison-land, I'm still fat fat fat." *sigh*

I've also been thinking about reasons to call *"goal"* and start T&M. Bad reasons:

1) wanting to eat something not OP
2) because my fat friends or jealous skinny friends tell me I've lost too much and need to stop
3) boredom

I've got a few more months. Hopefully I'll be acting from good reasons by then.

Corbie also talked about having sanity check friends to help you pick your goal weight. She suggested your doc, and friends who are a healthy weight without an eating disorder. If I expand that a little, to "friends who are not fat, not yo-yo dieters, and who don't have eating weirdness" I don't have anyone. Not a single friend or family member who I know well enough to know if they have weird stuff about food, who meets those criteria. Oh, and "eating weirdness" in my circle of friends includes eating disorders like bulimia, being on amphetamines and weighing 95 pounds, a friend who never eats anything green, a friend who has kidney issues + gluten intolerance and can hardly eat anything, a friend who is never hungry and forces herself to eat (and once took 45 minutes to eat a single Tostito), someone else not eating when stressed and dropping down to 72 pounds during exams, another having an anorexic mother and being raised all messed up about food/body image, etc. I think my best friend from 3rd grade would qualify, but she's currently living in Mexico and geographically isn't my best resource for feedback about my body.

So now I'm wondering—do I just attract people who are messed up about food because I'm messed up about food? Or is "food mental health" as rare as unicorns in our culture right now?

October 8: wearing a new skirt today

… and, um… I'm not quite sure how to say this. It's a, uh, medium.

Ack!

Went shopping with a friend last night and we spent HOURS at TJ Max. I got two knit dresses, like sweater dresses, that are all fitted and totally freakin' bombshell hawt. One of them I can wear now, and another in a couple weeks. 2 new skirts, one for now and one for a couple weeks. The "now" one is black on top, and then the lower half is gray/black ruffles. I'm wearing it with gray sweater tights and chunky-heeled librarian-ish shoes, and I'm kind of adorable if I don't say so myself.

I bought a bazillion pairs of tights in different textures and colors! As we lose weight thermo-regulation becomes a bit of a challenge. Also, I've decided I adore knee-length skirts. So between the two, sweater tights are kind of mandatory. Now I have a lot and I can liven up plain black skirts with pretty colored legs.

I also bought a bra. At home I have a wide variety of 40-D that I've shrunk into, and then out of. They gap. They're not good support. We picked out one 38-C that was deemed acceptable. It's a little tight, and it's weird for me to see my boobs all compressed like they're supposed to be and not vaguely cupped by a roomy sack. So I'm not wearing it today—I have to get used to the idea for a minute first. But I have it. A new bra that is smaller than any of the bras I own. (I have some 38-D pushup bras, but that's it.)

It was great having a friend to shop with. It's hard to see myself objectively right now, and I might have been scared of the knit dresses if she weren't there. Also, the bra fitting, well, I'm seriously out of practice. All recent bra purchases have been the fat-girl sports-bra type.

And I got earrings! They all fit.

October 11: I'm in the size 14s

My jeans... the 16s are in the Goodwill pile. The last couple weeks' losses have been slower, but I seem to be shrinking inches. Because the 14s fit like a dream now. It was 22 pounds in the 16s—that's a long time in one size!

Of course I'm having way too much fun with sweater tights and short skirts to actually wear the jeans, but at least I have them.

October 13: Holy hell I don't want to eat!

Tough day today, even aside from the drama on the boards. I woke up wanting to ask my best friend for a reality check—am I pretty enough to ask someone out? I've lost a lot of weight, but I'm still a few pounds away from overweight, I have a big belly, and things are a little saggy and lumpy here and there. I was having a small (large) crisis of insecurity.

Then I show up here, at the "supportive place," and someone is posting that a picture just like one I have up caused them "psychological trauma." Way to go, world—thanks for the pile-on!

So, that all sucks. I had a tearful insecure conversation in the alley behind work with my BFF. 90% about stuff I was feeling already, with some troll-frosting (lest you think the troll made me cry, which she didn't, I was all set to cry anyway).

Now I'm back in at work, it's time for my mid-morning soup, and I don't particularly want it. I'm all insecure, vulnerable-feeling, post-tearful, and screwed up, and I do not have the urge to shove a bunch of food in my face.

Is it possible I'm changing? This is a goodness. A very deep goodness. 65 pounds down and changing on the inside too...

October 14: My doc is adorable

I told him my knees crackle, and asked if I should be wearing flats more often instead of the heels I love so much. He said, "No, no—we'll give you some exercises for your knees. Let's get you all the attention you can get!"

Adorable man. He supports good shoes.

Also gave me a clean bill of health and took a new photo for my file. I guess my fatty-fat-fat face doesn't belong in there anymore!

He didn't know squat about MF, so I did some edjumacatin' while I was at it. He's a great doc, but didn't know this plan. But I'm walking proof. Oh, and he raised no objections to a goal weight of 135, the very top of "healthy" BMI for me. He just said "go for it" and was like—if it's what you want! So we'll keep tweaking as I get closer, but I got the seal of approval for the idea at least.

October 20: Well, it's all good news I figure

Still 100% OP. Down 67 pounds in 5.75 months, and I'm only 5 pounds from "overweight." New numbers from blood work: Cholesterol from 214 down to 151. LDL (bad cholesterol) down from 137 to 92. Vit D up from 15.5 to 69.6. My doctor is thrilled with me.

I'm smaller than the smallest I've been since about 1996–97. The skirt I could barely zip at my tiniest is a little loose now. I won't say things look as good as they did then—my belly is bigger than it was—but I'm smaller and weigh less. It's deep time travel now.

I'm pretty much just trudging along with the diet, doing my routine and watching my clothes get loose over and over and over. Shopping feels like a full-time job! I'm wearing pretty shoes and rocking the colored tights a lot. My legs I am quite happy with. Oh, and I'm down to a 36–C, which is a little ridiculous if you ask me. Not all of them, some were too small, but I found a couple which work now and why buy a larger size than you have to? If there's one thing I've learned it's not to buy something that fits properly anymore. Tight tight tight when you buy it...

I think size inflation has hit pantyhose as well. Have you noticed? When I put on a pair for which I'm smack in the middle of the suggested weight range, they have like yards of extra bunching up at the top of my thighs. When I put on A/Bs, or S/M, they fit great, even though I'm outside the weight range. I think pantyhose manufacturers have figured out women lie to themselves about their weight when they pick out a size, and have scaled them up a bit.

Anyway, hope everyone is having a lovely OP day. It works if you let it!

October 30: 70 down, 30 to go. Purgatory anyone?

Still 2 pounds away from "overweight" which seems insane. Still slim and lovely one day, horribly fat the next. Body dysmorphia, anyone?

Loving my smaller clothes—size 12 jeans fit comfortably and will be worn as soon as the muffin top recedes a bit more. Wearing an assortment of small, medium, and large—I just pick things out at random and buy whatever I can squeeze into. It's going to be baggy in a month anyway. I'm buying tights/pantyhose in S/M and A/B, which is kinda fun.

    This process feels eternal, and like how I live, and like purgatory. I feel like I don't have enough energy to do all I want to do. I want to go out to parties, or dancing, more than I do. But, I live on 900 calories a day and have my last meal around 8:00. Going out to a party that starts at 10 with a friend who won't want to go home until 2 is just plain hard. I'm super hungry by the end of it and just plain tired. So I feel like I'm waiting for the lush expanses of T&M for really kicking up my social life again. Which makes me a little sad, you know?

    If I hadn't read Corbie's great blog about goal weight I might be considering taking a break. But she said that when you've lost a bunch you feel all skinny because you're comparing yourself to fat you. But after a while, that comparison will recede and you'll be left still obese and dissatisfied. (I'm totally paraphrasing from memory of a couple months ago.) So, yeah, I can see that I still have a lot of fat on me. I want it to go away. So I'm hanging in here, committed to the plan, and just dealing with the purgatory feeling. 30 pounds. That's what, 3–4 more months? I can do it. I think I can even do it without losing my mind.

    Still OP. No breaks, bites, licks, or tastes. My food keeps getting simpler, with fewer recipes and modifications.

    I sure do miss being able to go into a restaurant and eat fried food until I'm full. *sigh*

    Hope you're having a wonderful day!

8 NOVEMBER

November 3: Been goin' out anyway

Who cares if I'm hungry and tired? Life is too short. So, after my whining last week, I went out to parties Sat and Sun nights (and shopping/massages with a friend Monday, and a movie last night with a group). Stayed out until 2–3am both weekend nights. I had shifted my schedule as much as possible, so I was only a few hours from my last meal by the time I got home. But I had a fantastic time and it does feel good to get out and play.

Also, I'm in my size 12 jeans as of last night. And panties—just threw out all the 8s and switched to 7s. Costco has six-packs of panties right now, so I have a stack of them in descending sizes—7s on top, then 6s, then 5s. I'm prepared for the next few months. Once I get to goal I'll have to figure out what works best with my new body and get cute ones, but in the meantime—functional Costco panties will have to do!

Cool mental shift this weekend. It just flipped in my head. I'm no longer counting up—20 pounds lost, 30 pounds lost, 60 pounds lost... I'm counting DOWN—30 to goal. It's a downward ticker in my head now. I feel a stronger relationship to the finish line than to the starting point. This feels very cool inside my head.

November 20: 75% Done. Yay for being a 100%er.

75 pounds down, 25 more to goal. Since April 28. Yeah, MF pretty much rocks.

I'm absurdly excited about my latest clothing purchase, which is a purple fleece-lined hoodie in a boy's size M (10–12). That's small, right? In my head it's small, when I'm shopping in the kids' section. The latest dresses are 10s, my jeans are slightly loose 12s, my tights are S/M, and it feels really good to be becoming a small person. *Really* good.

I want to make another plug for being a 100%er. It's been HARD the last week to stay OP. I've had PMS, and a lot of life stress, and too much success with the diet (you know, you start feeling good so you want to "take a break" or "relax for a minute" or sabotage yourself). I went to bed a couple nights ago just thinking about appetizer sampler platters from various cuisines. Fantasizing about the foods I miss.

But I stayed OP. I firmly believe the only reason I was able to is because for almost 7 months I've given myself No Other Choice Ever. Ever. There is no cheating, no BLTs, no nothing off plan. This has made my determination/commitment strong, and weakened my self-indulgence/addict. It has put me in a place where staying OP in the face of a hard week is possible. I can't imagine the struggle I would be experiencing if I let myself get "creative" with the plan, "listened to my body," or had a "little extra when I need it." What a living hell this would be, instead of just one of the hardest things I've ever done.

November 21: New kind of food dream

I love seeing how my subconscious has been dealing with food and this diet. I've been OP almost 7 months now, and I'm not having the "OMG I just ate a pizza—now what do I do?" dreams anymore. Last night I dreamed about whole wheat bread. I put some in the oven to warm up. Then I was looking around for a sheet that would tell me how many grams were supposed to be in a slice, so I could weigh a slice before I ate it. Then I remembered that the first week of transition was extra veggies, not bread, so I was going to wrap up the bread. Then I was looking for the transition guide so I could double-check the serving size on the veggies.

Yup. I've moved on to T&M food anxiety dreams. It's progress, right? *laughing* I'm still 25 pounds away, but my subconscious is getting ready.

November 22: It's not working

Well, I only lost a pound this week, well, for like 10 days, and so I'm pretty sure MF isn't working anymore, and I'm switching back to the drive-through diet because that was so working for me before.

Just FYI, in case anyone is wondering where I am, I'm trudging through the snow to get some fries. Or maybe ordering a pizza. Or Chinese delivery. Whatever. MF is broken.

November 24: Plan for tomorrow

I'm having a 4&2 day so I can enjoy dinner at my best friend's house. My last 4&2 day was September 4th for a wedding, but it's part of "my plan" for special occasions. And I think I'm calling tomorrow a special occasion. I normally eat my L&G for lunch, and I know I'd get too hungry if I tried to wait for dinner—so 4&2 if I want to eat real food at night.

5 ounces of turkey breast, no skin, and green beans without butter—I'm in charge of cooking them so I can do my portion separately. I'm bringing over my scale.

I figure, every couple months or so, it's nice to actually eat while at a meal with other people. Yay for turkey day!

9 DECEMBER

December 1: New pics!

I'm at 157, down 78 pounds. 22 pounds from goal (well, 7 pounds from my original goal!)
There's a second pic on my page.

December 2: Yup. Still hungry.

7 months and counting! I've been hungry for 7 months. I am getting to where this isn't really a complaint. The hunger was painful at first, a gnawing emotional thing with a heavy side of physical hunger. I had to take sleeping pills the first week or I couldn't fall asleep due to the hunger. Then I moved into the "occasional tough spots" time where it was mostly okay. I started embracing it a little, like learning to enjoy going to bed hungry.
I had a time where I was just incredulous. *Really?* I've been hungry for 6 solid months? *Really?*
Today, I post that it's been 7 months and 3 days. I've had physical hunger for significant parts of every single day, emotional hunger sometimes, and the *constant* feeling that "I could eat." I'm more detached. It's like, "yeah, so what? 7 months down. Maybe 3–4 more to go. Clearly it's doable. I've been doing it."
I've been 31 weeks OP, 79 pounds down = 2.5 pounds a week on average. My logged carbs average 82 for this entire period, which

puts my actual at about 85–88 with condiments. I'm burning fat, I'm in ketosis, and I'm still hungry, no matter what. There has been no combination of higher/lower carbs, larger/smaller L&Gs, 4&2 or 5&1, that has made me not hungry. I don't think I've been more than 20 minutes late for a meal more than a handful of times. My body is not fooled by ketosis—if it's burning fat for fuel it wants me to *know about it*. And yet, it's burning fat, and it's my friend for that, and I love it!

So, for those of you who think ketosis is helpful but not a miracle-worker, I just want to say *hang in here*. You can learn a new relationship to your hunger. You can even get to where you rewire your brain to experience hunger and want to go shop for cute tiny clothes instead of food. Seriously!

December 3: Denial. Crap was I in it.

I've been pondering some of the clues as to the depths of my previous denial.

- Handicapped bathroom stalls. I thought I just "liked them better." Really it was because I was so darned big that I was cramped in a normal person's stall. "Handicapped" was actually a fairly accurate word for what I had become.
- Pictures for personal ads. From time to time I'd decide to float an ad out into the world. I would use an old picture. In my head, this was because I just "didn't have any good pictures" recently, not an active intention to deceive someone. I didn't think "I'm too fat to show what I look like now." I thought "Here's a good picture from a photo shoot, and I don't have any recent shots that came out well."
- Acne. I would get a few zits before every TOM. I blamed hormones or something. Nope, recent experience suggests that was just due to diet and/or fatness.
- Indigestion. Gone. Was fat/diet.
- Creeping clothing sizes. I never once had the thought "wow, I've gone up a size." Every damn time I'd figure the line just ran small, or that I was just getting them a little roomy.

- I'm tired/I don't want to. Yes, I was tired. Because I was lugging around 100 freakin' pounds more than I should have been. I didn't just "not feel like" going to that party. I was worn out and killing myself just trying to live, and parties were not an option. Nor were a million other things.
- Overeating. I would think I was just going out for a fun meal with a friend. But it would be a fat friend, and we'd start with ordering an appetizer sampler platter before we even looked at the menus—basically "Just bring us everything you have that's deep fried." Then we'd order 3ish entrees for the table, plus bread/sides, and take home any leftovers. That's if we weren't at the all you can eat Korean BBQ. This was group overeating, a celebration of fat we could do together, giving ourselves permission to eat this way in public because we were together pretending it was normal. Somehow mysteriously since I no longer eat like this, this friend and I no longer manage to get together. I have friends who don't overeat who are still happy to get together at a restaurant with me and eat while I drink tea.
- My feet. No, I don't naturally have flat arches. I didn't require $500 custom orthopedic inserts because of some weird flat foot syndrome that kicked in during my 30s. I required them because I was fat fat fat and I was breaking down my own feet with that extra 100 pounds. Now I can wear whatever shoes I want.
- Sweat and smells. Guess what? I've become a pristine flower who wears the same clothes 2–3 times before washing them. I don't stink at the end of a long day. I will say nothing more about before.

So yeah. I'm trying to get clear about where I was and why. I need to remember, so I can stay on track to goal, and make a lifetime commitment to maintenance.

December 4: Entrenched *evile* thoughts!

Okay, "my plan" allows me to have a 4&2 day when I want to eat a dinner with friends for a special occasion. I've done it *twice* since I went to 5&1 in *June*. So it's not like I'm concerned I'm abusing the privilege, you know?

Tonight a friend is having a dinner at a steakhouse. An expensive steakhouse. So it would be a splurge for me to get steak + steamed veg, but it's not like it's going to break me or anything. And diet-wise I can be perfectly OP.

In trying to get okay with spending the money (on food, because clearly I've become okay with spending all sorts of money on clothes), I just caught myself thinking the evil thing:

"It will be a reward for making it to 80 pounds down."

Nonononononono! It's nothing of the sort. It'll be delicious, and I want it, and I'll do it because I will never ever in a thousand million years be able to properly sear a black-and-blue USDA Choice steak in my own kitchen at 1800 degrees, and it's exams, and it will be amazing. But my brain *really* wants to hook up "good food" to "treat/reward for good behavior" and I would like to stop it from such faulty nonsense.

sigh

Busted!

December 5: "Normal" food is starting to look pretty vile

(off plan foods mentioned below, but not eaten by me) 7 months on MF, 81 pounds down, I went out for dinner with friends last night to Daniel's Broiler, a (very) high-end steakhouse. I found myself fairly disgusted by what my companions were eating.

First of all, there were 6 women at the table (besides me) and all were overweight. I am fairly confident that if you went by BMIs they're all obese. And what they ate! Giant steaks with truffle fries and a massive bowl of ice cream for dessert. French onion soup. 4 baskets of bread eaten by 7 people, with *thick* layers of butter. A salad called "tomato and onion" which was covered in an almost equal amount of blue cheese and blue cheese dressing to the tomatoes/onions. A steak served with mashed potatoes and its *own gravy boat* of blue cheese sauce. Desserts of apple tart containing a few small apple slices, a crapton of pastry, a scoop of ice cream, and caramel sauce. Coffee served with a tray containing cream, sugar, and *whipped cream*. Really?

Now, my plate was a lovely work of art in my eyes. A steak which I cut in half and ate half of. I ordered it "no oil or butter, no sauce, dry spices okay, black and blue. No potato, no sides. What can you steam for me?" The answer was broccoli, so I said, "no oil, no butter, no sauce, but it's fine with me if it's a big pile of broccoli." My food arrived, I salted it, and while the broccoli was a little plain it was enjoyable. The steak was lyrically delicious and I can't really imagine it having been any better by adding anything else to it.

(And today for lunch I had the other half steak and a salad comprised of spring greens, tomato, and sea salt. Which I loved just as it was.)

For the first time, I truly, honestly felt not just not deprived, but like the food on my plate was exactly what I wanted on my plate. I wasn't jealous, I wasn't wishing to be someone who could "eat whatever she wanted." I wanted what was on my plate.

When I left, I felt as I always do. Not weighed down by carb-coma. Not guilty. Not torn by inner denial conflicts, because I assure you, I heard a LOT of conversation from these women about how they needed to lose some weight, and I guarantee you all was not resting easy in their minds. "Lord, make me good, just not yet." Well, I no longer have to feel that way. At least last night, my taste buds and soul and emotions and mind had all gotten on board with my new

Lifestyle.

Not a diet, yo. Lifestyle. Thank God for Medifast.

December 10: Who is that fat girl? Not me, certainly not.

Someone tagged a pic of me on FB. It's from an event in I think July, and I weighed 200 pounds. Oh, wow. I don't even know who that girl is anymore.

I untagged it instantly. I don't want people looking at my FB now to see that sad girl, eyes lost in big pillows of fat, round face like a moon.

I don't regret untagging it. I'm not okay with claiming that girl right now. But I do feel some sadness that my urge is to wipe away all evidence of the last few years. I had let things get Really Bad. They are Better Now. I am ashamed of that fat girl, and now that I've killed her I'm trying to destroy any sign that she ever lived.

I'm not sure if this is healthy, but it's what I'm feeling today. I let her exist here, in my photos on my page. She's here as a boogeyman, a terrifying ghost from the past, an ugly looming thing just out of sight that I'm running away from in the dark. I can't let her catch me again. She ate my entire life.

December 11: It's not tomorrow, but I'm starting to see the end in sight

I've got 18 pounds to my current goal. That's going to take 3+ months, depending on how much I slow down. But it's still feeling close. Today I'm wearing my size 10 jeans for the first time. I wear shirts tucked into skirts with a belt sometimes. I'm feeling pretty sassy and attractive most days...

Today, for the first time, I cut my MF VIP order to a smaller amount than replacement—the smallest amount to still get free shipping. And I pushed the ship date out as far as I could as well. I probably have 2 months of extra food stockpiled at home and at work, maybe more. I'm going to start reducing the stockpile some, with an eye for transition.

Kind of an exciting moment, in a quiet changed-my-online-order sort of way.

December 12: Got my first "anorexic" comment!

It was a future-looking one, not current, but still—it's got to be a good sign. I told a friend that I've got 18 more to goal, and she said I'll look anorexic by then. I told her that no, it would put me exactly one squeaky pound inside the "healthy" BMI range, rather than overweight. She just said the BMI charts were wrong.

I hear there's a stage coming up pretty soon when people start asking me if I'm dying. Can't wait for that one.

grin

ETA: I was not celebrating being called "anorexic" as a compliment. I was being ironic about how our culture sees a healthy weight as ill now.

December 13: Recovery isn't always polite

Well, I've been irritating someone with my blogs lately. (*Shocker*, right? Freya irritate someone? *Never!*) She was reacting to my description of several obese friends and what they were eating at dinner, and my saying I was disgusted by it. From what I understand of her perspective, she's concerned this might seem inhospitable/judgey to new people here. She didn't use the word, but I think I'm being accused of being fatphobic.

Well, it is judgey. It is full of judgment. But am I judging *them*, really? Hell no. I'm judging myself and the behavior I used to accept as normal. I used to eat way more calories in a day than was necessary for fuel. I used to go out with friends and eat piles of lovely greasy appetizers and fat-laden, carb-rich meals. And I would whine about how fat I was getting, probably at the same time.

This is *recovery*. I have been abusing food since I was 11, if not earlier. During times of great stress, I would "eat myself safe." Just keep eating until I felt better. Every tough change of school as a child, every rough breakup as an adult, and *wham* there go the extra pounds. I have an addictive relationship with food—I use it for the wrong reasons, and it's screamingly difficult to not do that anymore. I hit bottom with my morbid obesity that was incapacitating for the things I wanted to do in my life. I made a choice to do a diet plan that is humiliating. I have to eat space food packets, because my relationship with food is so broken I can't get back on track without serious rigid structure.

What happens in recovery? Well, if you're asking me, first off there's just a lot of pain. I really, *really* missed food at first. Then I just really missed food. I'd look at food porn. Dream about food. Talk about foods I missed. Miss foods some more. Cry, rage, have random inappropriate mood swings, and want to eat. Eventually, that started receding. I got a little better. I started feeling better. I learned more about how to cope.

I learned to shop instead of eat. I like shopping. Yes, it's a transfer addiction, but it's also necessary, so, well... I do what I can to keep it under control. I don't have cravings very often now, for old foods. Only when I really have stuff "up," and not always then. I can be around McDonald's food and it doesn't even smell good. I didn't even want to smell people's food when out at dinner last week.

And I did judge. It is normal, reasonable, and even healthy to move through a period in recovery when you find your old lifestyle disgusting. If someone were a recovering alcoholic, you would expect them to go through a phase when seeing people get sloppy drunk and make bad decisions would disgust them. You have to swing far away from something unhealthy first, before you can arrive at a lovely perfect balanced place of compassion for it.

I'm not there yet, about myself. Do I have compassion for my obese friends whose lives are limited by their health issues? Yes. Do I have compassion for anyone who is obese and can't stop eating? Yes. Do I understand perfectly, as a woman who has only been "not obese" for 10 pounds, and still has a large unpleasant belly? Yes. But I judge that behavior in myself. I hate the old pictures of fat me. I hate that I let myself get so out of control. I do not enjoy witnessing the same out of control behavior in my friends. And I don't even think that makes me an unsympathetic jerk.

I think it makes me a person in recovery. Working through an awkward stage of it, where I'm dealing with the wreckage of the past and getting more fully out of denial.

Recovery sucks. And it rocks. Loving and hating myself all at once is stressful and confusing and full of contradictory emotions. But I walk through it one day at a time, without comfort foods, and in my new size 10 jeans. Which makes it all worthwhile.

December 20: Might be time to start exercising…

I'm reluctant to say this, for fear it could bring back the rampaging hunger-beast, but I've been feeling pretty full for a few days. Like having a hard time finishing my L&G, and not really *needing* my pickles/cream cheese nightcap.

I'm a lot smaller. There's less of me to fuel, so perhaps I'm just not needing as much. There's also not a whole lot I can trim—when 7 ounces of tilapia feels like a lot, what can you do? Well, I can do 5 ounces of salmon, because then no healthy fats. I can skip the dill pickles. I can have lighter veggies like tomatoes instead of turnips. I've already quit eating maintenance bars for the most part, and I've been having more lighter meals like cocoa/shakes.

But other than that, I think it might be time to start figuring out what an exercise routine looks like for me. My body has been pretty willing to walk around a lot lately. Perhaps some actual sweating could come into my life, someplace other than the bathtub?

I feel like emotionally I could handle it if I exercise-stalled the scale at this point. Aside from my pouty ticker message, I'm really not upset by how little I've lost lately. I'm OP and I know it'll happen eventually. And exercise would tone up what's left, which I am in desperate need of.

Just thinking it over...

December 21: Naughty Santa costume—153 pounds

There was an event last weekend called "Santarchy" here in Seattle. It's several hundred people dressed up as Santa doing a pub crawl. It was a BLAST.

I ran around in a trashy Santa's Helper costume. I was thrilled by my energy—I was there for 8 hours, wandering the streets, in and out of bars, dancing a couple different times, and still felt great at the end of it. Hooray for MF!

December 22: What do you *really* want?

Okay, it's the holidays. Yes, there's a lot of food around. But seriously, who cares? Do you want to be fat for the rest of your life? Or do you want a thinner, healthier, happier existence right now?

This is a lifestyle change. There will be cookies and fudge and gravy in the world from now until the end of your life. Do you think it's possible, though, that you've already eaten enough of them for a lifetime? I have. I really have. After 8 months OP, I can tell you that I don't think about foods I miss in that longing way. I don't think to myself "at goal I can have that" (except for beets and Dave's Killer whole grain bread—and if either one is a trigger food I'll say goodbye without a tear.)

How did I get to where I can imagine a life without gravy and feel happy about it? By having a life without gravy, cookies, cake, fried food, or whatever else, *every damn day*. For 8 months.

A couple months ago I was thinking about just trying something, just having a tiny break, for one small meal's worth of binge. And I told myself, "If I'm not going to learn something new, how will I *learn?*" By which I mean, if I don't *try* it a new way, I can't *change* inside.

So I stuck it out. I have learned. I have changed. I keep learning and changing, and getting stronger and more powerful in my resolve every day. The rewards are immeasurable and a world of wealth unto themselves. I have attention from men, clothing I adore, a bouncy body that loves to dance and walk and skip and frolic (in pretty heels!), and *none* of my old obesity-related health issues. I'm remembering how to be happy, I sleep better, I spend more time with other people, I go to parties and events and have a great time. I would not trade this for *food*. Are you kidding me? Have you seen this cute body in this awesome dress? *laughing*

You don't need that lick of frosting or cookie dough. You don't need to eat like "everyone else" at Christmas. You don't need a glass of champagne at New Year's. You are here, on these boards, on this diet, because you *need help* to learn a new way to live and get control of your obesity. Accept the help. Stay OP. Learn to have a different life.

It's worth it. I promise.

December 22: Help me out here...

When you're scheduling dates with two intriguing men, that means you're officially "dating," right? Been so long since I dated that I've forgotten.

December 27: What's a successful meal plan look like, anyway?

Someone wants to know what the heck I'm doing, that I keep losing so well! The short answer is: stay 100% OP, all the time, day in and day out, because that's how you win the mental game. *No exceptions, ever.*

This means you have to plan ahead. When I leave the house at 2pm to go shopping with a friend, I take *all* the food I will be eating for the remainder of the day, even if I plan to be home in 2 hours. Seriously! I don't allow for any "mistakes" or "having to" eat off plan. I bring my food. I plan ahead. I make it happen.

In terms of food, I mostly follow the MF guidelines exactly. I have made certain small modifications for me, but I stick to those 100%. If I've decided that parmesan isn't a condiment on *my* list, I never eat it. Which again is key for the mental game. This shit gets *hard* sometimes, and if you never deviate from the plan, it's a thousand times easier to make it past the hard moments.

I was very successful on 4&2, and am doing well on 5&1. On 4&2, I stuck to the regular MF snacks, pretty much dill pickles for me, not the diabetic ones of yogurt/fruit.

In general, I don't worry about calories or carbs at all. If I follow the plan guidelines, it'll all work out.

I generally eat an oatmeal or hot cocoa/chai for breakfast around 9, and a chicken noodle (or other) soup at 10:30. I have my L&G at 1, which gives me good fuel for my afternoon. I'm too hungry if I wait for dinner. If there's a dinner event where I want to eat a meal at a restaurant, I still have my L&G at 1 so I don't get too hungry, and then have a 4&2 day. In the afternoon/evening it's 3 more MF meals at 3:30, 6, and 8:30. Then I have 2 dill pickle spears with however many healthy fats I get as cream cheese before bed. That's salty/fatty/fulfilling enough to tell my freaked-out self that I'll be able to sleep and make it through the night without dying of starvation. Ritual can be very helpful.

For L&G I mostly do really simple things. Plain grilled chicken on plain lettuce and tomatoes, with a little salt. Lots of grilled/roasted/steamed/raw. Egg beaters when I'm hungry. Not a lot of extra spices. I have a good variety of proteins from week to week, but I'll eat the same thing all week usually. I buy a big pack of something at Costco on Friday, cook it up, portion it, leave 6 portions in the fridge and freeze any extras. And then eat the same thing all week.

As I said I have the optional snack almost every day. It's dill pickles—the world won't end. I don't have much of a sweet tooth, so I'm not interested in the jello. I can eat celery if I want it instead. But, I do not have nuts, MF crackers/crisps, peanut butter, or any other high-fat/high-carb nonsense on MY snacks list. If I do, then I have to watch my daily carbs, and this diet is easier if I can grab whatever I'm in the mood for at that moment and not worry about my overall day.

My big modification of the plan is in the condiments arena. I don't count them. *But*, I have a severely truncated list that keeps getting shorter. As I find I can live without something, I just keep living without it. Like salad dressing. Who needs it? Not me. My current condiments list includes *only*: baking powder, dry spices, occasional extracts/soy sauce, better-than-bouillon, canned green chilis (only in MF eggs), and hot sauce (only in MF soups/eggs). That's it. What I'm doing is making up for the lack of counting by eliminating things that are carby/fatty.

I eat a whole lot of food, both MF and L&G, plain and simple. I eat on schedule pretty tightly. And I stay OP.

December 30: Warning—you can't make fat jokes anymore when you're thin!

I had a 3rd date last night with a charming man. He's a moderately fat man, because, well, that's how I like them. We were watching *Despicable Me*.

When the kids talked about how they liked stuffed-crust pizza, he said to me, "I like stuffed crust." I said back, "Shocking." It was delivered dryly, clearly teasing him, as clearly he likes his food.

As soon as it was out of my mouth I remembered I'm not fat anymore. Poop! As another fat person, it's a shared in-joke. It's clear when I'm fat that yes, I like stuffed-anything, especially if it's cheese it's stuffed with. As a thinner person, though, I just look like a jerk who's being critical of his weight.

Oh my god! Some of these new habits are harder to learn than others!

grin

Have a lovely OP day!

(And in case anyone is worried, he still took it in good humor, with a "I'll get you back, you sassy brat" twinkle in his eye. But I got lucky.)

10 JANUARY

January 2: Listening to my body?

For the last 8 months, I've operated on the premise that my body is a greedy idiot piglet, who got me up to 235 pounds with all that fake hunger and stories about how she "needed" this or that. I have learned *not to listen*.

Hunger doesn't kill me. I can go to bed hungry and sleep well. I can wait for my next meal during the day and still function just fine. I can live on 900 calories a day without a bite of sludge, for 8 months, and wow—yup—still here.

But I'm starting to think that there may be different voices in my body which have messages I want to listen to. Now that I've spent so long ignoring/squashing/starving the greedy piglet voice, is there something else in there I can now hear more clearly?

I've had a couple times recently when I found myself working to create a situation where I'd be out to dinner and so could have a 4&2 day. The first was when I was accidentally having less than half my lean (frozen shrimp weight issue). By the time I'd done this 3 days, I went to dinner with a friend and ordered plain steamed scallops and veggies. I was too fuzzy-headed to even figure out what I could tell them to cook it in, so I just ended up with plain steamed food. It was amazingly perfect-tasting.

The second was yesterday. On NYE, I overdid it. I ended up in the totally depleted crashed-out place where I couldn't get warm. It came from too much dancing too long after my last meal. Then yesterday evening, I was calling around looking for someone who wanted to go get dinner with me. I was thinking about Outback Steakhouse and a plain grilled steak and plain steamed broccoli.

Then I realized what I was doing. I was trying to find a way to have a plain, boring, lovely L&G. I was not fantasizing about any sort of sludge. I was seeking healthy food that's OP. And I know my body was still reeling a little bit from the bad place of the night before. So I had a 4&2 day without creating the excuse of a dinner out. I ate a lovely broccoli egg beaters frittata and felt much better.

So... Perhaps there's a voice in there that I can listen to. 4&2 is an acceptable option, and even recommended when one is going over the exercise limits for 5&1. I'm considering, tentatively, a truce with my body, where I try to figure out which voice I can listen to without sabotaging myself. I think one big clue is that the good voice wants plain steamed/grilled L&G, and not any of my bad-habit foods. I can also use external clues to assess which voice it is—if I'm freaked out emotionally, then I'll be less inclined to believe it's the good voice. If I know I've been pushing the limits physically, I'll be more inclined.

I have new limits. I've never done this extreme of a calorie deficit before. I find it weird to be discovering entirely new scary places I can put my metabolism into by overdoing it. *Look, Ma*, I found a new way to go off plan! I don't do formal exercise so I didn't realize I had to watch that 45 minutes!

Trying to find a good strategy for this. Dancing is one of my biggest NSVs, and rewards for my hard work. I'm not willing to give up one of my favorite celebrations of life. Going out late at night and seeing people I adore and being part of the social life of this town is another one of my favorite rewards for losing this weight—that's also not negotiable. On NYE I had pushed my meals back gradually during the day and was 1.5 hours later than usual with my last meal, and that wasn't enough.

I'll get it sorted out. Maybe with the help of a new friend—the healthy voice of my healthy body.

January 3: State of the Union...

- I'm getting the "how much longer are you going to be doing this?" concerned-face thing with increasing regularity. They're not quite yet openly attacking my staying in the weight loss phase, but there is some skepticism about it.
- I have hip bones that just stick out and stuff when I'm lying down. Ribs too.
- I am wearing a lot of size 8s. Size 8 The Limited pants. They're too loose. Also bought a bunch of things in Junior Medium, and Misses Small. (I started in a size 24).
- I'll be at goal in 11 pounds. This is messing with my head. *So soon!* I can't wait to find out if I drop my goal or start transitioning when I get there.
- I'm afraid to leave the comfort of 5&1/4&2, but I'm also excited for beets and Dave's Killer Bread (and Corbie's pumpernickel recipe!).
- I have *tons* of restless physical energy. I am always looking for something else to clean in my house, or something to go out and do. I am going to have to develop a lot of hobbies, *stat*, before I lose my mind.
- I love to dance!
- Dating rocks. Just FYI. It's the coolest thing ever. NYE dancing party date, then last night dinner and Tron (terrible movie) with guy #1, tonight board games with guy #2, next weekend guy #3 will be in town, guy #4 is trying to schedule a coffee date for this week. Am I bragging too much? It's my NSV and I'm going to celebrate having a busy calendar. Yay!
- I'm feeling very at peace with the idea that I'll have a food plan for life, that I can't be trusted to eat what I want, and that this is just fine with me. I like cute clothes and high heels and that men pick me up on the dance floor (literally, not pick-ups, but my date lifting me up to spin me around).
- I'm ordering just over $250 worth of food on my VIP orders, and pushing the date out to the last possible date. I'm reducing my stockpile. I'm utterly out of scrambled eggs and don't even care—my indifference to food keeps growing in really good ways.

- I've been wearing eye makeup every day for a couple weeks now. I like being all put together: cute clothes, "I bothered today" face, accessories, high heels.
- I'm so absurdly grateful for MF.

January 5: Why 100% OP is the *easiest* way to do this diet

There's a lot of enabling bullshit on these boards. I can tell you why. It's because many (most?) of us here are food addicts in some form or another, and we're in *various* stages of recovery or not-recovery. I want to put the idea out there for the newbies that you can choose which set of voices to listen to, and you can even make a different choice than the one you've made in the past.

When I started here, Chris was the featured blogger. I forget exactly how she phrased it, but very early on she pointed out to me (or maybe in one of her blogs) that if I really knew better than the John's Hopkins docs I wouldn't be so damn fat. Well, of course she said nothing like that, she was perfectly polite and gracious, but I got the message anyway—I do *not* know better, I am *not* capable of "tweaking things" or "listening to my body" in a healthy way. I needed to surrender to the plan, and I did just that.

I am so grateful that I chose that voice to listen to, instead of the ones that say "we're all human," "it was just one day," "have an extra bar if you're hungry," etc. Yes, I'm human, but that doesn't mean I can't follow a diet plan and learn to be different with food. Just one day? All we have is today. And I was *always* hungry—when would that one bar thing stop? I'd have never gotten into ketosis, I'd have never learned to sleep without having a snack before bed, and I most definitely would not have lost *ninety freakin' pounds*.

So why is it easier to be 100% OP? Mostly because it shuts up that whiny screaming entitled brat inside ourselves. Mine was quite sure we were dying. *Dying*. But the longer I told her that the 5&1 (or 4&2) was *all* she got, the weaker she became. Her arguments stopped having any sort of moral authority behind them, because, well, she was so clearly Just Damn Wrong.

Being 100% OP let me unhook the emotional/mental desire for food from physical hunger. If I knew that I was getting enough nutrition to prevent starvation, then I could ignore any physical hunger I was feeling. That left me free to feel the emotional/mental panic over losing the ability to eat for comfort. It left me free to work on feeling my feelings, and finding new ways to deal with them. It let me notice all the times I would have eaten for other reasons than to fuel my body.

Being 100% OP lets me stop having to make decisions and fight myself all day long. I don't have to ask if I "need" this or that. I just eat my scheduled food at my scheduled times. If I were to cheat at all, it would instantly open up a Pandora's box of "well, you had (fill in the blank) yesterday, why not a bite of this today?" It becomes a constant struggle. You can read the blogs/posts of countless people who went off plan for a special event or a vacay and their stories of how hard/impossible it was to get the MFin headspace back and get to goal.

So, give yourself a chance. If you don't try something new, you can't become something new. And wouldn't it be fun to try a whole new way of life? I can tell you that the view from here is quite good. And my size 8 skinny jeans make me feel like Queen of the World.

January 9: Love getting department store emails!

Macy's was in my inbox this morning, telling me about great discounts on *Juniors* clearance. Gone are the plus-size emails forever!

(Their mailing lists automatically adjust based on what you've been buying. It's neat!)

January 10: I cancelled my VIP autoship today!

I'm within 10 pounds of goal, and I have a *huge* stockpile of MF'in food. So, I'm going to stop bringing in new food until I absolutely can't stand doing without something, and eat down my apocalypse-stores. I'm starting to find old stale-tasting packets, as it's been 8 months and I'm sure some of this food has been sitting around that long. I want to go into T&M with a fresh supply of just the things I'm currently eating.

So, strawberry shakes (from my original free food/sampler pack), Swiss mocha, crab soup and all, it's going to go into my body. No more baking as I'm out of scrambled eggs. I believe I will survive this, though!

I've mostly switched to 4&2 it seems. I've just been doing too much dancing and staying up late. I keep blowing out my reserves on 5&1 with too much exercise, and it seems to require 4&2 that day and a day or two after. So, I'm just going to do 4&2 for a couple weeks and see if I keep losing—and also see if that lets me remain on an even keel physically with my current level of activity. I feel like after that 8 pound in two week whoosh I need to stabilize for a moment and let things settle out! My plan is to do lighter fare for my second L&G—salads, with shrimp or hard-boiled eggs.

January 10: This new face is like a super-power

I have all the personality and confidence of a long-time fat woman who refused to let it get her down. And now I'm a skinny beeyatch on top of it.

I *love* how many men I write to on okcupid write me back and ask me out. I've never had such a high percentage of interest. Medifast has opened up whole new worlds for me, and damn am I happy about it.

Also, I had no idea this face was in there! I was worried I'd uncover a wrinkly old hag when I lost my weight. Look at my "before" pics on my page and OMG you'll see what I mean—I had no idea I would end up looking like this.

Wheeeeee—this is the bestest NSV of all! Ladies, this is why we stay OP when it's *really really* hard! (Or, at least it's one of the possible reasons. *giggle*)

January 11: I'm investing in myself, right?

I bought a leather jacket last night. A tight, fitted, tucked-in-at-the-waist, adorable leather jacket. It's got slightly steampunk-esque hardware. I got boots that are perfect with it. Yes, it was all at the Rack so it was a bazillion dollars less than I *could* have spent on it. But it was still a lot for me to spend on one item of clothing.

Pretty much everything else I have has been coming from clearance racks at Ross/TJ Maxx/etc, as cheap as I could find things. I feel distinctly uncomfortable investing in an item of clothing that's not absolutely required, functionally, and is more expensive. I mean, $7 for capris is one thing. This is another.

And yet, OMG have I worked hard. I'm close enough to goal that even with 10 more pounds gone it will still be perfect—a tiny bit more perfect we think. (My enabling BFF and I, that is.) I feel like a rock star in it.

I was crossing the street by the post office and a cute guy in a car almost screeched to a stop to let me cross. He didn't have to. In fact, I've never seen someone stop that close to me, with me as far off to the side of the road as I was. He could have kept driving in perfect safety. And yet, he stopped, and smiled at me, and I knew it was the magic jacket.

January 12: Mystic Voodoo and Wishful Thinking

We've spent a lot of years feeling helpless, and looking for the magic pill to fix our obesity. Guess what? There's no magic pill. There's no surgery that will make it so you can't gain it back. There's no side-effect-free pill that will make you lose weight while eating sludge. There's no exercise program that will let you eat whatever you want and still be slim and lovely.

No. Magic. Pill.

But guess what? There is a plan that works. Medifast *works* if you let it. The plan materials are on this site at Success Tools: Eat Right. Print out the pdfs and memorize them. Carry them with you until you've got this nailed. Follow them to the letter, and you *will lose weight*.

Since MF works, there's no need for mystic voodoo and wishful thinking. You don't need to only drink shakes, or never eat more than 1 bar/day. You don't need to eat tuna 4x/week, or change your L&G every day, or eat the same thing every day, or tie your shoes backwards on Tuesdays. You don't have to eat meals or foods you don't like. You don't need to find creative ways to make this diet *harder*, and you don't need to *game it*. It works all by itself.

I think some of this stuff that circulates is just our masochism and self-loathing taking a new form. Surely we couldn't let ourselves have a nice bowl of MF soup and enjoy our meal! If we're going to lose weight, we have to suffer, and suffering is best done with another strawberry shake. Honest. I read it on the internets.

MF is a lifestyle change. It's a last-ditch save-our-lives intense change in lifestyle and eating habits. It's not a quick fix, fad diet, or instant solution. It's a boot camp way to change your relationship with food forever. So, since the plan works, and it doesn't call for any of this weird food-issue self-abusing nonsense, why not just do the plan as written? See what you learn?

January 13: My mama is proud of me...

She just gave me her fridge magnet. The one she's had since the 1970s that says "Nothing tastes as good as thin feels."

It's making me really happy to see it, knowing she's had constant struggles with her weight her entire life, and that this is representing for her that she sees I'm doing something different than what she's done. It means she believes in me. It means she sees that I've actually started walking with this idea, in a way she's never managed to.

Funny how a tiny little fridge magnet can express so much pride and support.

January 18: Size 6

Skinny jeans. Tucked into calf-high boots.
That is all. *happy grin*

January 19: One year ago today, I ordered me some *ugly-assed shoes*

Zappos just sent me an email to tell me that the shoes I bought a year ago are still available in my size, 8wide. Well, right now I wear 7.5 and no wideness is required. Also those are hideously ugly shoes which I wouldn't be caught dead in.

I bought them because they fit my custom orthotic shoe inserts. The ones that cost me $500. The ones I needed because I was breaking down my own feet with my out of control obesity. The ones that are now a distant memory.

Good morning, darlings! Hope you're having a wonderful OP day!

January 19: new pic of size 6 jeans, as requested!

Sorry it's a crappy bathroom photo at school, but it does prove that the Size Six Debut occurred! 144 pounds, down from 235 start.

January 23: fat goggles tell me I'm a big fat fattie

I'm 5 pounds from goal. I'm wearing a size 6. I weigh 140 pounds. My new hot man calls me "tiny." And I am having a REALLY hard time wrapping my head around it. I don't *feel* tiny, at all. I feel like a fat girl who is somehow magically managing to fit in smaller and smaller pants. But like somehow they're funhouse pants, so while they SAY a smaller number, really they swell up to fat size as soon as I'm in them.

And I'm pretty sure my belly is as big and flabby as it ever was. Seriously. It's huge. Just ask my brain.

I hear it takes a year or two for the self-image to catch up with the weight loss. It'll be good to lose my fat goggles eventually. Wowza.

January 27: Really lovely thought in my head just now

I just caught myself thinking, "I don't want to eat like a normal person. I want to dress like this."

Yes, it's a size 6 jeans + magic jacket day.

happy

February 13: So hard so close to the end! 3 pounds from goal...

Oh, this starts getting really hard so close to the end. It is *hard* keeping my head in the game. I feel like I'm back to 7 months ago, when it was a struggle, and not at all like the last 4–5 months which have been pretty peaceful by and large.

I'm tempted by fried food on menus, by the pizza in the car with me the other night, etc. I'm having food dreams. I had one where I ate a couple bites of some desserty thing, and I was like "maybe I should just transition if I'm going to get all sloppy like this." Last night I dreamed I ate a strawberry and drank half a full-sugar Coke. I was just feeling a big ole "screw it" in my heart.

3 pounds to goal. I think part of why it's hard is I don't know if it's going to take 10 days or 6 weeks to get there. You know, how much my body/brain will resist this. I am totally as scared to get there as I am annoyed that I'm not there yet. This journey has been FAST and completely life-changing. Part of me wants brakes. Part wants the accelerator. Part of me is already sad that soon I will stop hearing every day from people how amazing I look. What will I do when the constant stream of praise stops?

It's hard realizing I have to fight a mental battle again with this, when I had been just in the groove for so long!

February 22: 1 pound from goal—Transition starts 3/5

I've set a date to start transition: March 5. That gives me this week to get through TOM and hopefully take off this last pesky pound. Then the extra week. If I haven't dropped that last pound in the next 2 weeks, I'm starting transition anyway so I won't be obsessing (thanks for your advice, De!). If I rebound up and stay up with the extra veggies, I can always take them away again. But I feel it's time, and I'm going to go with that.

I *will* get to goal, or Chris will kick my azz. And we can't have that.

So grateful for these boards, and this amazing journey, and just thrilled to have been blessed with such success.

I realized over the weekend that no matter how long it took to lose my last pound, any beets I bought now would still be good in my fridge. It could take a month and those beets would still be delicious. That's how close to goal I am—beet-fresh close. *giggle*

Here I am to tell ya—100% works! Something else *might* work, but 100% *does* work. And *fast*. Just about 10 months to drop 100 pounds. Where else can you get that, and learn to treat food as fuel, all at the same time?

Hang in here, dears. Don't "tweak" it, don't BLT yourself off-plan, don't rationalize how you "need" this or that, or "have to" eat something to please someone else or be social. Just put your head down and stay OP, and you WILL get to goal. I haven't had a single bite of *sludge* in 10 months, and it's made me a different person. A better person.

I can't wait to find out what I get to learn in T&M.

11 TRANSITION

February 23: Goal.

100 pounds down, to 135. 9 months and 25 days.
Oh my God I actually did it.

March 3: Coolest NSV ever

Cooler than marking myself as "thin" on my OKCupid profile. Cooler than discovering that most bracelets are too big for my tiny wrists. Cooler than shopping in the Junior's section. Even cooler than size 6 designer jeans and size 8 Tahari suits. (Maybe not cooler than getting hit on all the time and having all this amazing zest for life, but hey—pretty darned cool.)

What is this ossum NSV you ask? Yesterday at the mall we walked past a GNC supplement store. Huge display of weight-loss products. I realized there is no weight-loss pill, powder, diet, plan, or magic beanstalk in the world that has anything to offer me. I'm 2 pounds below goal and ready to *stop* losing weight.

I can honestly say it never crossed my mind before that moment that I would ever be a person who didn't want to lose a few more pounds.

This is going to take a minute to get used to. *happy grin*

March 5: Goal measurements report

What does 102 pounds mean in terms of inches?

- Arms: –6
- Chest: –14
- Waist: –18
- Hips: –18
- Thighs: –8.5
- Total: –64.5 inches in 9 months 25 days.

W00t!

March 7: report from transition week 2

People have been asking me how it's going, and I've been reluctant to talk about it, basically because I'm conflicted as crap. I feel like I must be cheating or doing it wrong, because there are new foods and extra variables and I'm no longer exactly following a sheet of paper like a bible. But we all have to transition eventually, so I'll share what I'm doing.

Now, I want to say, I am in transition, and I didn't start the following until I was down about 85 pounds and getting way too much exercise for 5&1. For the first 8 months on plan I did 100% and did not deviate no matter how hungry I was, because I was unable to distinguish between mental/emotional hunger and physical hunger, and also, even if I was physically hungry I needed to learn I would not die if I stayed hungry.

Now I am working on listening to my body, within strict food-as-fuel guidelines. I may not have a structured exercise regimen, but yesterday I did spring cleaning housework for 7 hours. Had to be burning a calorie or two. So I'm sticking with what I've been doing for a couple months, which is to add in a couple ounces of lean protein if it's been hours since I ran out of food and I am body-hungry. Like if I was dancing from 11–1, and my last meal was at 8:15, I'd have a couple cheese sticks at 11. This did make the difference for me between crashing out unable to get warm and maintaining my body temp every day, so I've felt good about it.

My calories are running higher than the official transition plan, my carbs probably little low. Overall I'm keeping my calories just below the low end of my possible maintenance range. I am following the transition guidelines in terms of new foods, except that I'm doing dairy before fruit because I fear the extra sugar.

But I do want to say, I check in with myself constantly about the 3 ounces of chicken or 2 cheese sticks I might have. I check in to make sure it's not a "snackish" feeling, like I'm really wanting sludge. I check in to make sure it makes sense with my activity levels. I log every bite I eat and look at my overall day. And I am crystal-clear that I have the potential inside me to balloon right back up to where I started if I am not vigilant.

What would I recommend for someone else? Just follow the plan. For me, I have been unwilling to curtail my physical activity to stay within the plan as written, for only the last couple months. But that doesn't mean it's the best route. It just meant that I didn't want to watch a clock on the dance floor or in bed, and I was willing to accept the possible consequences of modifying the plan. I'm honest with my food log and weigh every morning, and if I start creeping up I'll know for sure I'm doing it wrong.

Fundamentally I just have myself to be accountable to, and I am the one who needs to be comfortable with my intake. It is very strange to be shifting my foods around, going down to 3 MF meals, etc. Today I'm having chicken vegetable soup for one of my L&Gs (I was doing 4&2 when I started transition, and am now at 3&2 + dairy + 1C veg), with Greek yogurt added in. I'm splitting the soup between breakfast and lunch, as I've eliminated a MF meal. It's disorienting to be having real food for breakfast!

I miss the comfort of space food. I miss the strict regimen. I feel uncomfortable and guilty about the extra food, the new schedule, the beets and butternut squash, the higher calorie count. When you've been eating 800–1000 for 6 months, and then 1000–1200 for a couple more, going up to 1450 seems like a massive uptick. I know it's below the low end of my possible maintenance range. I *know* I'm not gaining any weight yet. But I still feel like I'm doing it wrong, all the time.

sigh It is a hard change, leaving the weight loss phase. But I don't want to lose any more boobs and so here I am.

March 11: Transition: Target Practice!

I've had the most lovely mental shift around transition the last couple days. It did NOT hurt at all that I'm down 3 pounds in the 2 weeks since I hit goal. Body is not yet on board with stopping the losing! So, if body is going to be such an eager little thing, I'm going to have to throw more calories at it until it settles down.

This last week I've been eating around 1450 calories a day—between 1300 and 1493. I've decided to make 1450 my "number" for this week, and aim as close to it as I can. All of a sudden this became fun. It's not that I can't have more food, or I have to eat more food, or whatever. It's a giant calorie puzzle with a bull's-eye and my job is to try to nail it. Usually by throwing more eggs at it until it stops wiggling.

Next week I'll see what happens to the number when I add fruit and do whatever other adjustments I'm supposed to do for transition. I'll see what the scale says. And I'll pick a new number, and then keep trying to nail it.

No reason to see this as a chore, right? Calories in = calories out. The early part of maintenance is figuring out what that burn rate is, so you can eat the right number of calories. I read someone saying that if you're still losing, to add 100 more calories for a week and see what happens. So I'll fiddle the numbers up and down until I stabilize.

I'm so excited I've found a way to view this as fun. But really, what's not to love about 1450 calories? I'm warm a lot of the time, I get Greek yogurt in my chicken vegetable soup, and next week I will probably be leaving ketosis, hopefully forever.

Sure do love Medifast!

March 14: Transition: comes with some kewl stuff I barely remember

1) Keeping warm. I like do this. Naturally. Turned the heat off entirely when I went to bed last night. No shivering or whining in a couple weeks. *Seriously!*
2) Pooping. Nuff said.
3) Thinking. I feel like I'm at least 60% of the way to having my brain back. Longer focus, better concentration, more

drive. As I said about 5&1, the body would allocate calories for hunting down a bison, but inventing algebra was out of the question. I feel like my body is willing to allocate calories to thought again. Neat!

4) Tiredness. Okay, maybe this one isn't my favorite. But it's an interesting change of pace after the manic absurdity of the last many moons of ketosis.

Holding steady at 134 the last few days, which is perfect. Low of 132, goal was 135. I plan to maintain between 132 and 137, so I'm right on course. Doing pretty good at hitting my daily calorie goal. It's fun figuring out what my eating is going to look like now. At least at the moment, I'm still in the "cool game" mindset and not the "ZOMG leaving the safety of the womb" panic place.

March 14: Report from transition: trigger food identified

I'm going to go ahead and discuss the food because many people consider it on plan, as an optional snack, although I never did: nuts. Turns out I can't handle them. They are being ejected from the house in the morning—someone at work will be delighted to have the rest of the container.

Live and learn, eh? *sigh*

March 30: Why do we do 100%? Because it *changes* us

I was a 100%er during 5&1/4&2. I didn't cheat. I kept my head down, white-knuckled through the hard times, whined a *lot*, had crazy mood swings, went through withdrawal, missed the comfort of eating until I was stuffed, distracted and safe, realized I had a totally unhealthy relationship with food, and figured out I needed to treat myself like a junkie about food.

The plan was my lifesaver. Sticking to it 100% let me learn and change. I was thinking one day a few months in that a big bowl of my favorite greasy sludge would really make my stress all better. Then I realized, "how can I learn if I don't *learn*?" I had to experience something different in order to learn a new way to live.

So I stayed OP. Day after day, month after month. I lost 100 pounds in 9 months and 25 days. I've been maintaining below goal for 5 weeks—not a long time yet, but enough to discover some cool things about how I have changed.

- Fried food was my favorite thing. I ate a bite of a tater tot over the weekend and *spit it back out onto the plate*. It was so foul I could not believe I had ever wanted to eat that nasty mess. Yuck. I turned back to my plain hamburger patty and salad with pleasure.
- I prefer my food simple and clean. A curry is fine with each serving made with 1/6 of a tablespoon of oil, and a little nonfat greek yogurt to make it creamy. I don't need butter to enliven my life. In a restaurant, I genuinely don't want the sludge other people order. I want my lean and green, thank you. I still don't want any damn salad dressing on my salad, either.
- Some foods are triggers. I cannot eat roasted salted nuts without losing my mind. Other foods are not—I ate some bacon on Saturday and don't spend any time thinking about when I can have more. Same thing with bread—I'm indifferent to getting more of it. The slow experimentation of transition is a wonderful gift, because it lets me isolate which things are problems that I have to guard against, and which things are just foods I can choose to have sometimes. It lets me focus my vigilance on the real enemies: my triggers and my mind set, and not on food in general.

Would I be a person who orders L&G in restaurants now if I hadn't done 100%? I don't know, I didn't choose that road. But I do know that the road I did take involved not overstimulating my taste buds all the time. Not coming up with creative ways to mimic off-plan foods I was craving. Avoiding anything that I thought would be too stimulating/exciting/tempting. I didn't melt any cheese for the first maybe 4 months OP, because I knew I couldn't handle it. And last night? When I fried up a couple eggs in PAM, I considered adding cream cheese and decided I just didn't want it. Not that I couldn't have it, because I could have made that choice, but I didn't want it. I wanted my eggs plain, just a straight shot of protein.

That's the gift of the 5&1 boot camp. We have a chance, a unique opportunity, to find out what life is like when we don't act like junkies. I am forever grateful to MF for giving me that chance.
Will you take the chance offered to you today?

April 6: Report from Transition: Carbs are SO not my friend

I keep trying to incorporate the new foods, I really do. I'm not saying anyone else shouldn't follow the transition plan guidelines—I think they're great and sensible. I am just figuring out that my body is really unhappy if I follow them. Dairy is no problem, it doesn't bother me in the slightest. But fruit and grains? Not my friend at all. I look at the guidelines, and I know I'm supposed to be broadening my culinary horizons, but when I do I don't like how I feel.

It's not a carb addiction thing. Carbs don't make me want more carbs. But they do make me feel off-balance physically. I'm hungry right after eating, and stay hungry for hours. I end up trying to eat enough protein to get myself balanced out again, even when I'm not stomach-hungry. I'm just blood-sugar hungry.

I'm up 2 pounds in 2 days. I know I didn't eat 7000 extra calories in the last two days. I know it's the carbs hanging onto more water than not-carbs do. But I don't like how I *feel*.

This week, I have been eating a meal that is made with pork loin, pearled barley, apples, and turnips. It has a carbs to protein ratio of 2–1. Twice as many grams of carbs as protein. It makes me feel horrible. The rest of my food has a ratio of carbs to protein of between 1–2 and 1–3.5. Most of it has 3 times as many grams of protein as carbs. That food makes me feel great. It makes me feel *normal*. This ratio is easily achieved with a few ounces of "lean" and a substantial amount of veggies.

Medifast food is about even, carb grams to protein grams, as are the other-brand bars I've been eating. That's okay for the bars, but I don't feel inclined to do two in a row. I want to get a regular 3x protein meal in between. The flax crackers I like are almost even in their ratio. When I had been having quinoa, I had only 1/8C dry per serving, and I had it with enough protein that there was almost twice as much protein as carbs—49g to 29g. This was also okay for an occasional meal.

So there it is. Math. I'm starting to figure out my parameters for carbs. Keep the protein at an even level for an occasional meal/snack, and at double to triple for most of my meals. Then I feel good. Let the carbs outstrip the protein at any meal, and I get all wonky and don't feel in control anymore.

Yay for learning. I'm giving the rest of the barley/pork dish to my mother. Blech.

April 28: Mediversary!

OMG I just remembered today is my Mediversary! One year ago today I ate my first space food packet. Wowza has it been a journey.

Thank you, Medifast!

9 weeks since goal, today I weighed 135 (goal). Down 100 pounds from start.

So grateful...

April 30: Report from Transition: Mostly good, a little bad

I've been at or below goal for 9 weeks now. I'm a daily weigher. On just 2 days my weight has bounced back up to 136, and just 2–3 days at 132. Otherwise, it's 133–135, which seems grand to me.

My food routine is settling down. I eat close to my same 5&1 meal schedule. I have 6–7 small L&Gs depending on how long I'm awake. By "small" I mean most of them are in the 200-calorie range. I also have 1/2 ounce of flax seed crackers, and a protein bar or two. I was having Greek yogurt but I think I may be slightly allergic to it so I haven't had that for a few days and I am feeling better. It's a pretty simple diet still, but so far it's working well for me.

That's the good. I had a little bad last night. It was my last day at work, and I was beyond exhausted. I'd been talking non-stop all week training various people in various parts of my job. So much talking I was losing my voice. Pretty non-functional. Also a little freaked out about "what next?" as I'm now unemployed. It ended up being a bad combination, and I didn't have any reserves to call upon. I ate to stuff my feelings, rather than from hunger.

It's been a long time since I did that. Well, pretty much exactly a year since I did that. I only ate about 400 calories more than I normally would, but I had a couple extra Caramel Nut bars and I ate meals before I was hungry. I had that "out of control" feeling. I didn't like it.

This journey is for sure a work in progress. I guess one strategy would be not to get so completely wrecked. Another one would be to keep focusing on building better coping skills. Or just making myself go to bed instead of sitting up with the stress monsters—they made Ambien for a reason, right?

I know it's not about one day. 400 calories is nowhere near even putting a pound back on my ass. BUT, it's when one day leads to another and another, and the food choices stray off my food plan, and that's the bad road.

Maintaining vigilance and learning as I go…

April 30: The Different Flavors of Overeating

I was just thinking about how different they are.

There's the gradual "just a little bit extra" too-large serving kind, which I can do without even noticing I'm doing it. The difference between 200 and 300 calories does not mean the difference between "satisfied" and "omg why did I eat all that?" They both seem like normal small meals. But the 300-calorie meals will add up to about 600 extra calories *a day*, and before you know it I'm fat again because I put 4 ounces of pork instead of 3 in each of my meals.

Then there's the trigger-food kind. The Great Nuts Debacle of 2011, for example. It wasn't emotionally triggered, it was brought on by roasted salted nuts. Having them in the house caused me to lose my little peanut mind. There was no amount of "working through my feelings" that was going to avert that binge, because it was about the food.

Last night's was the emotional kind. The emotions were pretty simple—exhaustion, stress, a stubborn stress-based refusal to go to sleep, and boredom. I needed to be comforted. I went for the wrong kind of comfort.

I need to have strategies to deal with all of these and more, I'm sure. Help me out here, dears—what other kinds of overeating are there?

I'm perversely impressed by how *many* different ways I've found over the years to abuse food. Takes talent, right?

May 3: Your Pants Get Tight, You Eat a Little Less

Reporting from T&M here...

I'm feeling better, as the scale is cooperating. I'm back down to 134 this morning. I had been up to 137, which is the upper limit of my 132–137 maintenance window. I dropped my calories a few hundred for the last 3 days, and got my carbs down between 71 and 87. Obviously I didn't lose 3 pounds of fat in 3 days—it was water bloat from letting my carbs get up too high. But it feels good to see the number go back down.

I'm staying on my "reeled in" plan until I see 133, and then I'll go back to having dairy (pending allergy testing) & protein bars.

I am very excited about this. I was eating too much, I gained, then I ate a little less, and I lost. I didn't have to dive back into 5&1, and I *did not let it go unchecked.*

This may be the coolest innovation in the history of man. All those skinny people have known about this forever, but it's news to me. Your pants get tight, you *eat less.*

Wow. Stunner, right? Who knew moderation was even a remote possibility for me around food?

May 7: Guilt—Is it Helpful?

I can't tell if guilt is serving me well or ill at this point. Before I started MF, I had the whole "no, I shouldn't be eating this let's do it in secret" guilt/shame thing. On MF, I had "anticipatory guilt," where I could imagine how crappy I'd feel if I let myself and all of you down by eating off plan. Pride kept my spine straight, as it were.

Now, in T&M, I still have a lot of guilt. I feel guilty when I eat. I always feel like I could be eating less, or I could have waited a little longer. I feel like my carbs "should" be lower. I feel guilty over this food or that food, even though they're part of my plan.

It's not like this isn't working, right? I got up to 137 for a minute, and reeled myself back in, and 5 days later I was down 6 pounds to 131. It's not like I can't course-correct. I've been maintaining in my range of 132–137 since I reached goal February 23rd.

So why do I still feel guilty? Is it helping me to not eat fatty/carby/sugary things that aren't on my plan? I'm not sure. Surely

I could avoid those foods without feeling like a bad person much of the time I'm eating anything at all.

I'd love your thoughts on this. Do we need the Guilt Monster to lose/maintain?

May 18: Obsessed with Food Everywhere—Even in Fiction

I'm totally laughing at myself today. I'm reading a novel, and in it, the main character is hungry but doesn't get to eat. I am all concerned about when she'll be able to get a snack. I'm more concerned than when someone is shooting at her or she's about to be strangled by a zombie.

I do the same thing when watching TV—I hate it when characters order food in a restaurant and then ignore it to argue with each other. "People, can't you argue and eat at the same time? Get a grip—that's lamb curry in front of you!"

About halfway through the weight loss phase on 5&1 I was out to dinner with friends. They ordered fried appetizers, and left some one the table. There was fried food that survived an entire meal and no one was going to take it home. It hurt me to walk away from it.

Thankfully time and practice has made this easier. I can ignore the food that is "not for me" on a table, even if it's going to end up in the trash. Still not my favorite thing, but not painful any more. It's been hard to learn not to treat my body as the trash can for that unhealthy food.

Got any quirky ways your food obsession plays itself out? Surely someone's got something sillier than me being all worried about whether the heroine is going to get her supper.

May 19: Me and my short memory—science FAIL

[I'm 3 months post-goal, in T&M] Well. It had been 2 full months since the Great Nuts Debacle of 2011. I got cocky. I thought, "Gee, I don't even like peanuts. I mean, I really don't like them. What could it hurt if I got the rice crackers with the peanuts in them for a little extra protein? I had rice crackers last week and managed them fine—1/2 ounce at a time, no urge to binge."

It hurt. So now I've gone and lost control over a food I *don't even like*.

Lame.

sigh

It's logged, they're gone, and every day in T&M is a new day. I'll stay on track tomorrow without nuts.

Even peanuts. *Lame!*

May 21: Report from T&M: Pretty Damn Good, Actually

3 full months since goal. My last post was about failed science, so I thought I'd reflect on what's going *right* in T&M.

- I weighed 135 this morning, my goal weight. I have not gone above my maintenance window (132–137) at any point.
- I have tried a variety of new foods, including processed snacky things, and have only found one that's a trigger. For the rest, I've eaten one or two bites of things occasionally to try them, and not needed to have more.
- I've learned that my body doesn't like sugar at all, and I don't enjoy the taste of it anymore.
- I've learned to manage grains in small doses that don't trigger cravings.
- I can order healthy food off a menu.
- I log everything I eat.
- When I get close to the upper end of my maintenance window, I gently course-correct, dropping my carbs down below 100, and the weight disappears in short order.
- I am eating small L&Gs 6 times a day, with some protein bars and whole grain crackers, and my body is quite happy with this diet.
- I have a simple system for making 250-calorie meals, using the Sparkpeople recipe calculator.
- This feels possible. Maintaining feels possible. I'm so grateful.

KEEP IN TOUCH

Thank you for reading *Suddenly Skinny Day by Day!* To stay in touch, please visit facebook.com/SuddenlySkinny, Twitter @SuddenlySkinny, or SuddenlySkinny.blogspot.com.

Made in the USA
San Bernardino, CA
01 December 2012